HEALTH CARE OF THE ELDERLY

HEALTH CARE OF THE
ELDERLY
Strategies for Prevention and Intervention

Edited by

Gari Lesnoff-Caravaglia, Ph.D.
Sangamon State University
Springfield, Illinois

Volume I, Frontiers in Aging Series

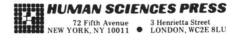 **HUMAN SCIENCES PRESS**
72 Fifth Avenue   3 Henrietta Street
NEW YORK, NY 10011 ● LONDON, WC2E 8LU

RC952
H4

Printed in the United States of America
0 987654321

Library of Congress Cataloging in Publication Data
Health care of the elderly.

  Bibliography: p.
  Includes index.
  1. Geriatrics. 2. Aged—Medical   care. 3. Aged—Medical   care—United
States.
  I. Lesnoff-Caravaglia, Gari.
  RC952.H4   618.9'7'00973   LC 79-19192
  ISBN 0-87705-417-7
  ISBN 0-87705-486-X pbk.

For

John H. Keiser
P. Douglas Kindschi
Robert C. Spencer

whose generous administrative support and
understanding materially advanced
the academic pursuit of gerontology

CONTENTS

7

CONTRIBUTORS

ELAINE M. BRODY, M.S.S.A., Director, Department of Human Services, Philadelphia Geriatric Center, Philadelphia, Pennsylvania

ALEX COMFORT, M.B., B.Ch., D.Sc., Consultant, Geriatric Psychiatry, Brentwood Veterans' Administration Hospital, Los Angeles, California

SUE COX, Director of Volunteer Services, Hospice, Inc., New Haven, Connecticut

HERBERT A. DEVRIES, Ph.D., Andrus Gerontology Center, University of Southern California, Los Angeles, California

BENNETT S. GURIAN, M. D., Massachusetts Mental Health Center, Boston, Massachusetts

GARI LESNOFF-CARAVAGLIA, Ph.D., Associate Professor, Gerontology; Director, Gerontology Program, Sangamon State University, Springfield, Illinois

ERIC PFEIFFER, M.D., Professor of Psychiatry, University of South Florida College of Medicine, Tampa, Florida

THEODORE R. REIFF, M.D., Professor of Medicine; Director, Institute of Gerontology and Geriatric Medicine, University of North Dakota, Grand Forks, North Dakota

ETHEL SHANAS, Ph.D., Professor, Department of Sociology, University of Illinois at Chicago Circle; Professor, School of Public Health, University of Illinois at the Medical Center, Chicago, Illinois

VIRGINIA STONE, R.N., Ph.D., Professor, School of Nursing, Duke University, Durham, North Carolina

DONALD M. WATKIN, M.D., M.P.H., formerly Director, Nutrition Program Staff, and Special Assistant to the Director, Office of State and Community Programs, Administration on Aging, Office of Human Development Services, DHEW, Washington, D.C.

INTRODUCTION

Were someone to propose that a particular segment of the population be excluded from medical treatment or be deliberately left unserved by the health care professions, indignant voices would be raised in outrage. Nonetheless, the exclusion of older persons from such care and services, conducted however quietly and subtly, has occasioned almost no protest whatsoever.

Neither Senate hearings nor open pleas have ruffled the academic complacency of those responsible for the training of health care professionals in the field of gerontology/geriatrics. The greatest concession the topic has received in some medical circles has been the occasional generation of pseudointellectual arguments as to whether or not geriatrics is a specialty.

In the meantime, the number of aged persons in our society continues to increase, bringing with it the increased need for geriatric health care. The primary response to these needs, thus far, has been either to permit older persons to cope as best they can while ascribing their ill health to the processes of aging, or to institutionalize them.

There are a number of reasons why the treatment of older persons in the United States is unpopular and regarded to be unnecessary. The principal factor is attitude. That ageism operates in the medical field as well as in the larger society is not surprising, since health care personnel, brought up in such a cultural milieu, do not bring special perspectives to their chosen field. Nor are their attitudes counteracted by education or training. Generally negative attitudes reinforce the indifference toward the aged, resulting in the lack of educational training and provision of services.

In the United States over 80% of the medical school graduates take up to 5 years of postgraduate specialized training; almost none of this is devoted to geriatrics or even to a cursory overview of the field of aging. With few exceptions, nurses also receive only negligible training in this field; most nurses who are currently employed in long-term care facilities and other health establishments serving older persons have developed their capabilities in the practical school of experience—that is, on the job.

Medical care of the elderly means more than prescriptions and diagnoses, and requires the consideration of persons in their total complexity within particular environments. The concept of treating the whole person must take in this broader perspective in order to be effective.

Furthermore, few medical schools are so organized as to offer opportunities for interprofessional training and collaboration. Equally lacking is a multidisciplinary approach to teaching about health care for the elderly, their problems, and society's responsibilities with respect to these problems. The result is that not only are health practitioners poorly informed about the health care needs of the elderly, but they are equally uninformed about the competencies and roles of other professionals in providing services and influencing policies that have direct bearing on the lives of the elderly.

Geriatric medicine has not received the stature it should have in this country's medical training programs. Through such discrimination in medicine, it has been exceedingly difficult to attract physicians-in-training to work in this area, and, subsequently, few geriatricians are available as role models in medical school facilities. Furthermore, there is little appreciation for the fact that geriatric medicine actually provides an excellent environment for the in-depth study of human disease.

In addition, older persons have not been very visible in our society. They are either hidden away in their own homes, in institutions, or in segregated communities. The older persons medical students are apt to see, and these only in a few medical schools across the nation, are ill and probably have been suffering from a variety of ailments all of their lives. The healthy aged are not seen by physicians, and they are only beginning to be seen by the larger public as well. The myths and stereotypes that currently abound may in the future be dispelled by the ever-increasing numbers of older persons in society who will insist upon equality of treatment.

The present negative view of the processes of aging and of the aged has also prevented medical personnel in the United States from regarding the ailments of older persons as treatable. There is not the search for causes in the illnesses experienced by the elderly, and unfortunately, there are still notations on death certificates giving the cause of death as "old age."

Autopsies are not performed at the same rate as they are in the case of young persons, nor are accidental deaths carefully investigated. The emerging issue of abuse of the elderly may finally begin to deal with the unexplained falls, fractures, concussions, burns, etc. that appear on death certificates as having occurred in the home environment, as well as in institutional settings.

In the United States the basic professional curricula of the core professions providing medical care to aging patients (family practice, internal medicine, psychiatry, and nursing) contain little or nothing specific to working effectively with the specialized aspects of care of the aging. The often-aired argument whether geriatrics is a specialty or not, in the face of greatly increased requests for medical services, is as practically based as were medieval discussions of how many witches could dance on the point of a needle.

The emphasis in American medical training has been on the treating of acute illnesses: on rapid cure and release of the patient to the home with the resumption of an independent existence. The treatment of older persons is in diametric opposition to such a pattern. The older person who comes to medical attention is usually suffering from one or more chronic ailments and will have a prolonged hospital stay with little or no dramatic change in condition, with possibly a gradual decline or even death. Should there be some improvement in the patient's condition, a discharge will very likely be to an intermediate care center, a nursing home, or greater dependence upon existing family. Such a change in the nature of medical practice is insufficiently recognized in the United States.

In part, the lack of provision of medical care for older persons hinges on what has been described as a tug-of-war between the integrationists and separationists. Medical schools appear to be divided on two main issues.

1. The segregationists argue that the elderly have specific medical problems requiring special attention, thus the need for a separate department of geriatric medicine in medical schools.

2. The integrationists see no need to single out the treatment of the elderly in our medical schools because aging is a developmental phenomenon, and there are no diseases that strike the elderly alone. They feel that instructions about the medical problems of the elderly can be integrated into conventional course work.

It appears that gerontological/geriatric education in the United States is still in the wishful state. There is much dialogue with respect to what ought to be done, but from the vantage point of aspirations, rather than of accomplishments.

The implications of neglect for health care delivery are very real. Older persons experience more acute and chronic diseases than the younger population. Psychopathology in general, and depression in particular, increase with age. Suicide sharply increases with age in white males; and while a little over 10% of the population is over 65, this group uses 27% of the health dollar. Yet little attention is given to the promotion of health and the improvement of the quality of life for the elderly, both of which would work to alleviate the complications of chronic disease and depression that frequently result from inevitable losses and isolation.

In an attempt to bring constructive action to bear upon the health problems of older persons and to stimulate increasing awareness of the need for gerontological/geriatric education, the Sangamon State University Fourth Annual Gerontology Institute, held in the spring of 1978, was dedicated to health care of older persons with an emphasis upon strategies for prevention and intervention. Papers selected from the presentations at the 1978 Gerontology Institute are included in this volume.

ACKNOWLEDGMENTS

The Gerontology Institute is an annual cooperative effort developed by the Sangamon State University Gerontology Task Force, whose membership includes agencies and organizations in the state of Illinois with interests in gerontology/geriatrics. The Task Force is chaired by the Director of the Illinois Department on Aging.

Cosponsors of the Gerontology Institute 1978 included the Illinois Department on Aging, the Illinois Office of Education, Roche Laboratories, and the Department of Family Practice at the Southern Illinois University School of Medicine.

The development of the Gerontology Institute as an integral part of the Gerontology Program is largely due to the assistance and guidance of Francis F. Pyne, Dean of the School for Health Science Professions, and Larry E. Shiner, Dean of Academic Programs at Sangamon State University.

The coordination required during preparation of the manuscript could only have been effected through the patient and untiring efforts of Candace Corrigan.

Gari Lesnoff-Caravaglia

Part I

MEDICAL CARE OF THE ELDERLY

The advantage of being an aging society is that we are forced to reassess our entire value system and, specifically, to reflect upon such values in terms of attitudes and behaviors. This is particularly relevant to the area of medical care.

The presence in our society of increasing numbers of older persons is leading us to alter gradually the meaning of medical care. It is no longer sufficient to examine, diagnose, and prescribe. Attention must be paid to the recipient of such services.

Such attention must include recognition of the close relationship among psychological state, social milieu, and biologic condition of the person. Even routine aspects of medical care, such as history taking, assume a new dimension when the patient is an older individual.

Such a reassessment of medical care and medical practice can only lead to optimism, for such alteration of caring procedures is to the advantage of all persons, regardless of age.

Chapter 1

BIOMEDICAL ASPECTS OF AGING AND THEIR RELATION TO GERIATRIC CARE

Theodore R. Reiff

Aging has been a very poorly understood phenomenon. It has been poorly understood by the public in general, and since the medical profession is really made up of members of the public, I think that the misunderstanding also has applied to the medical profession.

A story told to me by an elderly patient illustrates how poorly understood older persons are by their physicians. It is the story of the 78-year-old man who goes to see his physician and proudly announces that he is getting married. His bride is a beautiful 28-year-old girl, and the two of them have decided that they wish to have children. He asks his doctor for advice. The doctor thinks for a moment, but not much more than a moment; then he turns to the patient and says, "Well, why don't you take in a boarder?" The patient thanks him and goes on his way. The doctor hears nothing for about 3 months. When the patient returns, he joyously announces that his wife is expecting their first child. The doctor congratulates him, but secretly congratulates himself, thinking what a wise physician and counselor he was to give such good advice to his patient. As the patient is leaving, the doctor turns and says, "And by the way, how is the boarder?" The patient looks at him and says, "Oh, she's pregnant, too."

If there is any humor in the above it is because it upset our expectations about the needs and also the abilities of older persons. I think we have all seen this lack of knowledge and the resulting prejudice in our own fields and disciplines, regardless of what they are.

STUDYING THE AGING PROCESS

If we are going to talk about aging and understand something about aging persons, we first should look for a definition of aging. I would propose that the best way to think of aging is not in terms of chronological *real* time, but rather in terms of a series of processes or events that take place in real time. For example, we know that aging is not unique to living things. Everything ages. Engineers talk about the aging of a bar of steel. By aging they mean a series of physical or chemical processes or events that take place in time. Another reason it might be better to think of aging not as the passage of chronological time but in terms of processes or events, is apparent in the true story of microorganisms that have been found frozen in the Siberian tundra by Soviet scientists. They brought them into the laboratory and put them into a warmed-up culture medium; the microorganisms have begun to metabolize, grow, and reproduce. By special methods utilizing radioactive isotopes dating or, more recently, by measuring the amounts of dextrorotatory and levorotatory amino acids, we can determine how long ago those organisms became frozen. Some of the calculations reveal that this freezing occurred as long ago as 400,000 to 500,000 years. The question, then, is how old are they? Are they 1 or 2 days old—that is, the 1 day that they had been growing and metabolizing before they became frozen, plus the day they have been growing in the laboratory now—or are they half a million years old?

That is a moot point, a semantic problem; but if you define aging in terms of a series of processes and events, the problem disappears because during the years the organisms were frozen, they were not undergoing biologic and chemical processes that we identify with life. And since the science fiction of today is the reality of tomorrow, human beings of the future may very well engage in interplanetary and possibly interstellar space flight by freezing or suspended animation of some type. In fact, freezing experiments have been done, not just with unicellular organisms, but with multicellular organisms. They have been frozen, not only for hours or days, but for weeks and months, then subsequently thawed and continued their life processes.

Yes, it has already been done with some forms of life, and there is no theoretical reason it cannot be applied to human beings as well.

In order to alter the rate of aging, we must know something about the biologic mechanisms of aging. Thus, some of the leading so-called theories of aging will be reviewed here, followed by information regarding how that knowledge could be applied to our handling and thinking about problems of aging in human beings.

Genetic Error Theory

One of the earliest theories of aging, and a very interesting one, is the error theory, which was largely developed by Dr. Leslie Orgell, a Fellow at the Salk Institute in La Jolla, California. Almost 20 years ago Dr. Orgell postulated that aging may be due to an accumulation of genetic error in the deoxyribonucleic acid (DNA) of cells as they replicate. The idea was based upon the fact that the genes of our cells, which reside in the chromosomes, undergo self-replication prior to cell division, before a new generation is produced. And they replicate themselves very well with good fidelity.

Suppose that with each replication only 99% of the DNA molecules that make up the genes replicate correctly; thus there would be a 1% error with each cell division, with each generation. That error would tend to be cumulative, so that by the end of 10 generations of cells one might have almost 10% error in the DNA; that might be just the amount of error that would prevent further replication and result in death of the cell line.

In fact, there has been good physical and chemical evidence of DNA error. Electron microscopy and certain physicochemical techniques have revealed that indeed there is error in the DNA: As it replicates, a certain amount of it makes mistakes.

The error theory of aging was held to be quantitatively a very important theory until a few years ago, when another discovery shed some doubt on its importance. That discovery was that residing within the nuclei of cells are specific endonuclease enzymes that, incredible as it may sound, are capable of correcting the error by "snipping out" the error portion of the molecule, allowing for insertion of the proper DNA gene sequence. And the endonuclease enzymes are themselves very efficient (more than 99%). Even if there were a 1% error in DNA that accumulated with each generation of cells, 99% of it would be corrected, leaving only a .01% error with each generation, or 1 part in 10,000.

Nobody knows, however, what the critical amount of error is that would preclude further cell replication. Thus, although the discovery of endonuclease activity has altered the quantitative importance of the error theory of aging, it has also opened a new field for correction of genetic errors that cause disease. For instance, sickle-cell anemia is caused by a genetic error in the DNA that codes for the production of hemoglobin, and an abnormal hemoglobin is produced. If we could identify the abnormality in the fetus or even earlier, perhaps in the gamete (the germ cell), and introduce a corrective endonuclease, we might be able to correct the genetic error that makes abnormal hemoglobin, and prevent the development of a disease. This could be accomplished for a whole host of other diseases that have genetic components or counterparts.

Free-Radical Theory

A second theory of aging, one that has some possible therapeutic implications or preventive implications, is the free-radical theory. Free radicals are molecules that are highly reactive chemically because they have either a surfeit or deficit of electrons, or they have electrons in higher energy states. It is known that radiation is one of the things that produces free radicals. In fact, chemists use radiation to produce free radicals and cause an acceleration of chemical reactions.

About 15 to 20 years ago, Dr. Denham Harman, who is Professor of Medicine and Biochemistry at the University of Nebraska College of Medicine in Omaha, postulated that aging may be due to an accumulation of free radicals in tissues, and that these free radicals, being highly reactive chemically, go around doing a lot of unwanted damage. Harman did not simply hit on this idea while he was sitting in an armchair thinking about it. Rather, he based his theory on experimental information: Included in that information was the previous observation that radiation given in sublethal doses will shorten the life span of entire populations of experimental animals. Some of the initial work was done with drosophila fruit flies. There were no immediate deaths, but just a general shortening of life span; Harman thought that perhaps the mechanism was the radiation, producing free radicals.

Radiation consists of high-energy photons that hit molecules; this energy can either raise an electron in a molecule to a higher energy state or knock an electron completely off. Either way, an electric charge is produced on the molecule, making it more reactive. The free-radical theory of aging has also received some possible support by virtue of observations in humans who have been exposed to radiation.

As we know, the world's first nuclear-fission bombs were

exploded in August 1945. Actually the first bomb was exploded in July 1945 as a test, but the first use was made in August over the Japanese cities of Hiroshima and Nagasaki. In addition to the hundreds of thousands of deaths caused outright by the explosion, large numbers of the population in both cities who survived were exposed to sublethal doses of radiation. In 1945 the United States established the Atomic Bomb Casualty Commission to study the effects of radiation on the survivors. The work seems to indicate that some of the parameters of aging in the Japanese survivors have been accelerated. There is an increased incidence of lenticular cataract formation, which is an aging change. Certain other changes in the integument of the skin and hair also parallel those noticed in aging.

The problem, though, is severalfold. First, the evidence is not conclusive, and second, there is no baseline information on the affected population. It was largely a civilian population, and any medical records that existed in doctors' offices and in hospitals on these people (i.e., the biologic information on them) was all destroyed in the explosions. If it had been a largely military population, there would have been a central repository of records, presumably at some other place in Japan, where we could have obtained some baseline data. For instance, the United States has all its medical record information on military personnel in a huge storage area (called the Military Personnel Record Center) in St. Louis, run by the General Services Administration (GSA).

However, in the early 1950s an opportunity, if one can call it that, presented itself to the United States to get information on a controlled population. At that time the U.S. exploded the world's first fusion bombs in the Marshall Islands in the western Pacific. On March 1, 1954 the U.S. Navy, which was in charge of the experiments, set up at Bikini Island what was called a fail-safe experiment. It was said there was absolutely no chance of danger to human life and that radiation could be carried no further than a radius of 50 miles from the center of the explosion. Thus they evacuated all of the islands for a radius of 50 miles from the epicenter of the explosion. The day came: It was said to have been a "beautiful" explosion, and the expected things happened. The ships in the lagoon nearby were either sunk or capsized, and the nearby islands were incinerated with all their flora and fauna. Islands further out had varying degrees of radiation exposure, and everything was going very nicely; the meters were clicking off the radioactivity, and everybody was getting the information they wanted, when something rather unexpected happened. There was a shift in the winds of the upper atmosphere, and the fallout, which consisted largely of the highly radioactive strontium 90 and radioactive iodine, began to be carried much further than the 50-mile absolute upper safety limit that had been declared. Fallout was carried over 80 miles; then it began to descend in a fine radioactive ash over the island of Rongelap, which was inhabited by South Sea natives.

Before the Navy realized it, the entire population had been exposed to about 175 roentgens in air, a sublethal but highly significant radiation dosage. The Navy quickly evacuated the island, and since that time (1954) the Rongelap natives have been studied very carefully. Rongelap had been a protectorate of the United States, having been ceded to it by the United Nations after World War II. The U.S. was thus responsible for the health of the inhabitants of the island, and in that capacity had collected a good deal of baseline biologic and medical data on the islanders. In fact, a good deal of what we now would call ecologic information had been compiled on the flora and fauna of the island. Here, then, is a population on which we have good biologic and medical information before a uniform radiation dosage, who have now been followed for over 24 years, since the exposure.

The children from the island were obliged to undergo thyroidectomies to prevent the development of cancer of the thyroid, since it is known that iodine concentrates in the thyroid gland to make thyroid hormone, and the glands of children are particularly susceptible to developing malignancy from radiation. The thyroidectomies have largely prevented the development of thyroid malignancy.

Unfortunately, strontium is a chemical that is very similar to calcium: it is a divalent cation that goes to bone like calcium; unfortunately, it binds even more tightly to bone than does calcium, and its biologic half-life is very long. How many of the children, now adults, are going to develop osteogenic sarcoma and other bone malignancies as a result of the exposure to the radioactive strontium 90, we do not know. Unfortunately, you can't remove people's bones as you can their thyroid glands.

We might say, "Well, what's happening with the people from Rongelap?" We don't know yet: 25 years is not enough time. But it is expected that by the year 2000 or thereafter we should have, for the first time, a very careful study of a population of humans whose biology and medical status were known before radiation exposure and who have been followed assiduously ever since to observe the effect on aging. We hope that this will provide some answers.

All of this is very interesting, but why discuss the free-radical theory of aging at such length? The answer is that something can be done about it, maybe. Dr. Harman has been doing experiments in which he places in the food of animals from the time they are born, materials that inactivate and bind up or prevent the absorption of free radicals. He has found that the life span of rats can be increased by significant amounts by the simple expedient of giving these materials to the animals, or to their pregnant mothers.

More recent experiments have involved pigs, the reason being that pigs are very close to humans from a biologic point of view. Immunologically their systems work very much like humans. Harman has been able to increase life span significantly in pigs. This is very significant, and you might ask why we don't immediately start adding this stuff to the foods we all eat. But as close as pigs are to human, humans still aren't pigs, and one cannot apply information from one species to another so quickly.

There are a number of reasons this experiment has not been done with humans. Think of studying a human population from the time they are born, and having children eat this material in the food continuously throughout their entire lives. One would have to check them at periodic intervals; do tests on them; have them stay on this diet when they go away to school, to college, and after they get married. It is hard enough to get children to eat regular food, let alone food with additives.

There is thus a practical logistic problem, and then there is an ethical problem. Would it be fair to subject children to this diet or these additives, which we do not think would be harmful, but we are not sure?

Then there is a third problem. Aging research has until recently been considered (and still is in many areas of government and our society) to be low-priority research. An experiment like this would be very expensive: It would require great expenditures for personnel, for equipment for testing, and for following the people.

Another problem is that if the experiment were started today, the results would not be available until 2050 or 2060. We wouldn't know for a lifetime how effective it was going to be.

Thus for many reasons the experiment has not been started, but all is not so black. It may be possible, and even now people are beginning to study the effects of these additives on human cells in tissue cultures. It may be that we can find some answers in the not too distant future. First, do these additives lengthen the healthy life span, and second, are they nontoxic?

Hayflick Phenomenon

A third theory of aging also deserves considerable attention because it is not only fascinating, but it has tremendous implications. The Hayflick phenomenon, named after Dr. Leonard Hayflick, who was Professor of medical microbiology at California's Stanford School of Medicine, where most of his work was done, and more recently is at Children's Hospital Medical Center, Oakland, California, where he is a gerontological investigator.

About 18 or more years ago, Dr. Hayflick became very interested in human tissue culture. He started some experiments that to some extent repeated work that had been done at the turn of the century by Dr. Alexis Carrel, a French surgeon and scientist who was working at the Rockefeller Institute in New York City. Carrel had the "crazy" idea that if you supplied the right environment to tissue, perhaps you could keep it growing indefinitely, even forever. He put heart connective tissue cells from chick embryos into tissue culture, and he supplied the right nutrients, the right temperature, the right acidity, the right amount of oxygen; he took away the waste products. The cultures grew, and they grew very well. About half the time, however, after a certain period of time had elapsed, it seemed that one half the cultures would die out. The other half kept growing pretty well. The ones that died out he blamed on his technician, claiming that she used improper technique, or that she sterilized the glassware improperly, or that she put the solutions together incorrectly. She said he was wrong, but this was before the days of women's liberation so the results were attributed to "technician error."

This work initially generated great interest; people reasoned that Carrel had shown, theoretically at least, that we can live forever if supplied the right environment and the right nutrients.

After awhile people lost interest in Carrel's work because nobody ever lived forever. Thus until the 1950s there was very little work done in human tissue culture, and Hayflick began some of it. Other investigators were also involved in this work; still others have continued in even more elegant ways than Hayflick.

Hayflick's results were much the same as Carrel's, although he used a slightly different tissue line. He used connective tissue fibroblasts from the lungs of aborted human fetuses. Hayflick found that the cultures seemed to grow quite well for about 50 generations, (50 cell divisions), after which time about half of the cultures would die out while the other half would keep growing.

He went a little further than Carrel did, though. He examined very carefully the morphology of the cells that kept growing, and he found something very interesting. Instead of the diploid number of chromosomes (23 X 2 or 46) that is characteristic of human cells, some of the cells exhibited either triploidy (23 X 3 or 69) or polyploidy in bizarre numbers (100 or 150 chromosomes); and some of the cells had multiple nuclei. Some of the cells began to get very large and to grow very wildly; as the reader may recognize, he noted that the cell cultures that continued growing for more than 50 generations, had undergone malignant transformation into cancer. His published work caused great excitement. Observers reasoned that Hayflick had discovered the cause of our limited longevity, why we live to only three score and ten: We either run out of cells, or we develop cancer; and we die of cancer.

Indeed Hayflick at first believed that to be the case; but then he and others calculated the amount of tissue that could be produced if, from the time you were a fetus, your connective tissue cells were capable of fifty replications.

Not all cells in the body, however, undergo 50 replications. Some have more, some less. Connective tissue cells are in fact rather primitive cells that form the basis for differentiation for many other cell lines. There is even some evidence that smooth muscle cells may be derived from connective tissue cells. Hayflick calculated that if a fetus had connective tissue cells capable of 50 generations of normal healthy cell divisions, the mass of tissue produced would be enough to last 150 to 175 years. The implications of this are staggering: There is perhaps a cellular limitation to our longevity, but we never come close to reaching it. In fact, from the connective tissue point of view, we may be living to only 50% of our biologic cellular potential.

Another very significant discovery has recently been made: There is in brain tissue a substance as yet unidentified, but probably a peptide, that is capable of causing more than double the number of healthy cell divisions in a cell line. By adding this substance to tissue cultures, researchers have increased the number of cell replications from 50 to over 100. The implications of this are very significant.

Hayflick and other scientists have expanded upon this research. One of the things they have been studying is the number of cell replications as a function of age of the organism from which the cells were taken. It was indicated earlier that fetal connective tissue cells were capable of 50 replications. In additional studies, connective tissue cells were taken from a 10-year old child; it was found that the child's cells had about 40 replications remaining. Cells were then taken from a 30 year old, and these cells underwent about 30 replications. Cells taken from a 70 year old were found to undergo about 20 replications. Extrapolating this curve of cell replication potential as a function of age of the organism from which the cells were taken to the point at which it reaches zero replications, this point turns out to be about 150 years; this further confirms Hayflick's calculations of the amount of tissue that could be produced.

Current Thought

Since the aforementioned experiments, some preliminary work has been done on the numbers of cell replication in children with a rare disease known as progeria. Progeria is a condition in which a child, who at birth looked absolutely normal, begins to undergo some unusual physiological changes as he approaches puberty (age 8 to 10 years). The child will start to have graying of the hair, and a male may start to undergo some balding. As such children approach puberty, their second teeth may begin to fall out, and their gums recede. They start to develop lenticular cataract formation, and their skin starts to wrinkle; in short, they begin to look and act like old people. Most of them die in adolescence of the diseases commonly found in old age or in older persons. Recently a few have survived into their 20s because of advances in supportive medical care.

Hayflick and others have studied a few people with progeria. There have not been many studies of this disease because, fortunately, there are not many people with progeria. Researchers found that the progeric 10 year old might have only about two or three cell replications left. In other words, it appears that there is a family of cell replication potential curves, and it may be that what limits the life span in progerics is the limitation of cellular replication potential.

Some interesting work is also being done on diabetes and in other diseases, indicating there may be limited cellular replication potential in various disease states. Some evidence suggests that some of the normal-appearing siblings and parents of progeric children may have cellular replication potentials on intermediate lines between that of the progerics and the normal. The implications of this work are extremely important, among them the discovery that it may be possible to increase cellular replication potential by certain methods, such as adding brain extracts. This has tremendous potential significance with regard to possible CNS effects on longevity. It should be noted that this work has been done in vitro and not in vivo, i.e., in the living organism.

Dr. Nathan Shock and his colleagues at the laboratories of the Gerontology Research Center in Baltimore, Maryland (now the laboratory of the National Institute on Aging), have been studying aging effects on human beings by bringing older persons into the laboratory at periodic intervals and measuring many physiological functions. This experiment has been going on for more than two decades with almost 1,000 subjects, and they have been studying a whole host of organ functions in relation to age. Maximal organ function occurs, not surprisingly, in the 20s; by about age 30, organ function begins to decline. From about age 30, when there is 100% of maximal in cardiac function, pulmonary function, muscular function, kidney function, bone strength, nerve conduction velocity, in practically every organ system that has been studied, there is a decline of about .5% to .75% per year from the maximum. Even the immune system shows a significant decline in function with age.

One might assume that this is what does us in: We lose organ system function, so that by the time we are three score and ten, we lack sufficient organ system function to keep us healthy. It is not true, however, the reason being that we are born with a great excess of function. We have two kidneys when we could get along fine with one or less than one. We have two lungs, but could live quite well with only one. Thus we have such excesses of strength and capabilities that we do not start to get into physiological trouble until we are down perhaps at the 35% or 40% level. The decline in organ system function is not doing us in, then; that will not get us into trouble until we are well past a century, unless superimposed disease further reduces function.

Quite possibly it is largely atrophy that does us in. Atrophy refers to the decrease in functional ability and also the decrease in size of an organ with disuse, with lack of proper stimulus or exercise. The opposite of atrophy is hypertrophy, the increase in function and size of an organ with proper stimulus and use. Atrophy and hypertrophy are universal biologic phenomena. They occur in every organ system ever studied. Cells actually decrease in size with atrophy; there is a decrease in protein production and RNA synthesis. The opposite occurs with hypertrophy, in which RNA and protein synthesis increases in the cells. If some of the further decline in organ system function with age is indeed due to atrophy, it is a very optimistic bit of information, for something can be done in relation to atrophy.

The decrease in physiological function due to age may be altered; atrophy may cause an increased rate of decline of function, and hypertrophy may cause a decreased rate of decline. In other words, the prevention of atrophy due to disuse, by proper utilization and stimulus of the body and its organ systems, may enable the body to continue functioning above the level at which continuation of living becomes difficult. (See Figure 1-1.)

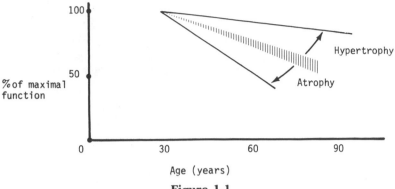

Age (years)

Figure 1-1

It would be well to discuss briefly at this point the potential for the extension of the healthy human life span and also some aspects of the role of immunocompetence; that is, the competence of the immune system in aging in relation to premature morbidity and mortality.

The immune system consists, in part, of certain types of white blood cells called lymphocytes. The two main types of lymphocytes are the B-cells and T-cells. The B-cells are capable of making antibodies when stimulated by an antigen, which is usually a foreign protein or substance that will cause the production of an antibody, which is also a protein. The antibody inactivates or binds up the antigen. For example, when given a tetanus shot, an individual is given killed tetanus bacilli, tetanus toxoid. The protein in that material stimulates the B-cells to make antibodies, which then can inactivate tetanus toxin, should the person ever get infection with tetanus bacilli. This prevents one from getting tetanus, as the B-cells make antibodies.

It has been found that with age there is a moderate decline in the functional ability of the B-cells. It has been found that with age there is an even more profound decrease in function of the T-cells. The T-cells are quite remarkable in that they have the capability of recognizing self from nonself. They can differentiate foreign cells from the body's normal cells; they can recognize invading organisms or altered normal cells. When they do recognize them, they destroy them, so they are called killer cells. The T-cells help to protect us against cancer. There is evidence that at least several times in the course of a life, a person may develop cancer cells, but does not get clinical cancer because the T-cells recognize the cancer cells as being foreign. Once such recognition is made, the cancer cells are destroyed, and the development or growth of cancer that could spread to other parts of the body is halted.

In older persons, however, the T-cells show a significant decline in function. Recently it has been found that there may be ways to enhance T-cell function, that is, to stimulate the immune system. Certain chemicals or materials may be introduced to enhance the immunologic function of T-cells.

Other recent information indicates that the immune system is capable of being psychologically conditioned. Some very important experiments in this connection were done at the University of Rochester School of Medicine in Rochester, New York. The researchers gave rats an immunosuppressant drug that depresses T-cell function. One such drug, called azathioprine (Imuran), is given to patients who have undergone organ transplants. Why? An organ transplanted from another donor is foreign tissue; the T-cells will recognize it as being foreign and attempt to reject and destroy it. That is what causes a graft rejection. The doctor gives the recipient an immunosuppressant drug, which suppresses the T-cells just enough to prevent rejection of the grafted organ, but not enough to suppress it completely so that the patient dies of infection. Azathioprine, as suspected, reduced T-cell function in rats. Upon removal of the drug, their condition returned to normal.

Before giving the rats the azathioprine, the researchers had given the rats another substance, saccharin. Saccharin proved to have no effect on T-cell function. It would not be expected to have an effect, since saccharin is a harmless sweetening agent in the dosage used. The T-cells, then, were normal when tested with saccharin; but when azathioprine was given, T-cell function declined. Once the azathioprine was withdrawn, the T-cells again returned to normal. This procedure was repeated several times.

Subsequently a mixture of azathioprine plus saccharin was administered to the rats. The function of the T-cells declined again, which was expected since the rats were getting azathioprine. This procedure was also replicated many times with the same result.

A new experiment was then devised. The rats were given saccharin alone, and the T-cell function declined. The saccharin was taken away, and the T-cell function returned to normal. The researchers had instituted a Pavlovian conditioning experiment, and had conditioned the immune system of the rats to respond to an agent which should have had no physiological or pharmacologic effect.

More recently, a number of reports in the psychiatric literature have surmised that one of the things that can suppress the immune system in humans is psychological depression and withdrawal from activity. With treatment of the depression, immune function seems to improve. In other words, it has been established biologically that the immune system can be psychologically conditioned and, very importantly, that psychological factors may influence immunocompetence.

A number of other factors can also have such an effect. Undernutrition or malnutrition can negatively influence immunocompetence. The CNS apparently can have an effect on the immune system. The implications of this are extremely important. Why?

UNDERSTANDING MORBIDITY AND MORTALITY IN THE VERY OLD

What is causing older people (i.e., those aged 80 and over) to get sick and to die? We know a great deal about cause of death in Americans. There is a virtual "epidemic" of heart disease or arteriosclerosis. This information is based on very careful postmortem examinations of people who have died in their 40s, 50s, and 60s. However, there is very little reliable mortality information on people over 70 or so. This is because very few postmortem examinations are done on older people.

If an individual in the mid-40s were suddenly to drop dead, everybody would want to know what happened. An autopsy would be done, and it would most likely show that the person had a cardiac arrest with a cardiac arrhythmia; cardiovascular disease would be the primary cause of death. If the person were 80 and dropped dead, not only the family, but even the doctors would say that he/she had died of old age. A postmortem examination would not be requested. The final rejection of the aged in our society is that we are not even interested in finding out why they die. As a result, there is very little scientific information on the cause of morbidity and mortality in the very old.

At the University of North Dakota as well as in Baltimore, there have been attempts to obtain morbidity/mortality statistics on very old people dying in nursing homes. With permission from the families, postmortem examinations were conducted. Unfortunately, the data collected were not sufficient to be statistically valid; but some pilot information is developing. Such investigations have suggested the very interesting possibility that the causes of death in the very old are far different from the young. It would appear that the leading causes of death in the very old are: (1) infection, (2) pulmonary emboli, and (3) malignancy. This is very interesting, because the first and the last, infection and malignancy, are very closely related to the decreased immunocompetence referred to earlier.

The second cause of death, pulmonary emboli, is largely related to physical inactivity. Pulmonary emboli result from phlebothrombosis (blood clots in the veins), usually in the lower extremities. Veins have valves that prevent backflow of blood. Thus the blood can only flow forward, because its backward pressure on the valves closes the valves. One of the things that helps return blood to the heart is muscular movement in the lower extremities, which puts pressure on the veins and thus propels the blood forward to the heart. Muscular activity and exercise keep blood flowing; without it, the blood just stagnates in the veins. Blood that is not flowing freely tends to clot or to undergo thrombosis. Thus one of the contributing factors in phlebothrombosis is inactivity of the lower extremities, that is, lack of exercise.

When the blood thromboses in the veins, there is the danger that some of the clot will break off and be carried first to the heart and then on to the lungs. Blood clots in a major pulmonary artery (pulmonary embolisms) can cause death if they are big enough, or numerous enough. And, in fact, it is a very frequent, underdiagnosed cause of death in older people.

The leading causes of death in the very old appear to be related to inactivity, atrophy, and lack of function; psychological depression may be playing a role in this inactivity. If this is so, it is again optimistic news, because it is something that we can do something about. In the future we may be able to do something about arteriosclerosis and about the cardiovascular diseases and strokes that are killing younger persons, but the morbidity and mortality of people who are over, say, 75 or 80, may be even more preventable or reversible than we think.

Role of Water

Another fact important in the clinical treatment of older persons is that total body water decreases with age. The embryo is 90% water. The fetus is 80% water, as is a newborn child. The amount of body water continually decreases, so that by adulthood it is down to about 70%. The amount of water continues to decrease with aging, so that when we reach our 70s the percent of body water has decreased to somewhere in the 60s.

Of what importance is this information? It is of great

importance when we consider the function of water in the body. For one thing, water acts as a diluent for administered drugs; it is the volume of distribution in the body for many drugs. Thus if there is a lesser amount of water in the body, and the same dosage of drug is given to an older person as would be given to a younger person, the concentration of that drug will be increased because there is less of a volume of distribution. The concentration of drug may increase to toxic levels, because the effects of drugs are related to their concentration. This means that the dosages of drugs that are dissolved or diluted by the body water must be adjusted in older persons. Unfortunately, it is not the usual practice to do so.

People think very little about adjusting pediatric doses. Whoever would think of giving a two-year-old child 10 grains of aspirin; and who would think of giving digitalis to a child in the same dosage as would be administered to an adult? Nobody. In geriatrics, nonetheless, we seem to have lost sight of the fact that the physiology and pharmacology can be different.

The development of pediatrics was beset by the same kinds of trials and tribulations that geriatrics is now experiencing. Perhaps 50 years ago, the attitude of internists was that children were simply little adults and that no special knowledge was required for treating younger patients.

One of the ways in which pediatrics established itself, so the story goes, was in Europe in the latter part of the nineteenth century. One of the children of the crown prince apparently got very ill, and he was getting worse. All the physicians were called in to tend the child. All the internists were stroking their beards and making one recommendation after the other, and the child kept getting worse and worse. Someone went to the crown prince and said, "Why don't you call in the Kinderarzt?" The crown prince said, "The Kinderarzt? A child's physician? What's that?" And the man replied, "There's a fellow who practices as a Kinderarzt over here, and he's supposed to be pretty good." But the other doctors said, "No, No, No. There's nothing new; there is no such thing as pediatrics; we don't need that." The crown prince, however, decided to bring in the Kinderarzt anyway. And, as might be supposed, the child got better after the pediatrician came in. The way pediatrics got established in that country was that the next day the crown prince said, "There is now a specialty of pediatrics." It is uncertain that we will have to proceed in the same way with geriatrics, nor is it clear that we need a separate specialty. What we do need is all physicians trained in principles of aging and geriatrics, with some geriatricians to act as consultants, investigators, and educators.

In any event, treating older people requires different approaches to drugs, and it is important to bear in mind some of the physiological reasons. We have to think differently about administering medication to older people. Some of the reasons relate to the decrease in organ function.

Many drugs are excreted by the kidney. If kidney function decreases with age at a rate of .5% to .75% of the maximum per year, then someone at 80 may have 40% less kidney function than a person much younger. If you are going to give to that person a drug that is excreted by the kidney, the rate of excretion of that drug may be decreased 40%. Thus if you give the same daily dose that you would give to a younger person with 100% normal kidney function, the medication will build up to approach toxic levels in the system, since it would not be excreted. This is exactly what has often happened in administration of certain digitalis preparations: The kidney function of older people was not taken into account, leading to frequent toxic reactions from digitalis.

The same is true of other drugs—some that are metabolized in the liver and other organs, some that are excreted by routes other than the kidney, such as the respiratory system. Since all these things change with age, the pharmacology of older persons has to be different.

At this point another example of the importance of water in the body is pertinent. Water is a very interesting substance. It has a high specific heat (1 calorie/g/°C), which means a lot of heat is required to raise its temperature. Thus you have to add 1 calorie of heat to raise the temperature of 1 g of water 1°C. Other substances have much lower specific heats. A bar of metal or steel has a lower specific heat (it does not require as much heat to raise its temperature). As an example, put 100 g of iron into a glass, and put 100 g of water into another glass; then place both glasses on the dashboard of a car in the summer for an hour. If you then touch the iron, it will burn your finger. Put your finger in the glass of water; it will be warm, but it will cool the burn. There is the same amount of each substance, so why does this occur? The reason is that the specific heat of water is higher and can absorb more heat before its temperature goes up.

As mentioned earlier, the body composition is 70% water in a younger and mature adult and only perhaps 60% in an older adult. This means that the older adult has less of a thermal buffer. The older adult cannot tolerate as much sun in the summer, because he/she does not have a thermal buffer of body water sufficient to prevent raising of body temperature and thus will develop hyperthermia more quickly than someone younger. Conversely, a 70 or 80 year old cannot tolerate the cold of a North Dakota winter: He/she will develop hypothermia much more quickly than would a younger person, because he/she lacks a sufficient reservoir of heat stored in the body water to prevent lowering of the body temperature.

Government officials did not take into account the danger of hypothermia when, in the interests of conserving energy, they asked us to lower the room temperature to 66°F (19°C). It is uncomfortable, they said, but it will not do any harm. But this is not true for older people. A younger person has enough heat stored in body water, enough competence of body thermal regulatory systems, to withstand environmental temperatures of 60–65°F over a long period of time without getting into trouble; this is not so for many older people. An environmental temperature of 66°F for a person in his/her 70s, 80s, or 90s, may be lethal. It may result in hypothermia.

Dr. Robert Butler, Director of the National Institute on Aging, recently had a conference in Washington, D.C., to point out the danger of hypothermia in older persons. It is insufficiently recognized, not only by the lay public, but by physicians as well. Hypothermia can be prevented, and it can be treated.

The different physiologies of older persons require a different approach to the management, treatment, and the recommendations for their living.

Role of Immunocompetence

An important difference in the physiology of older people in relation to their health and survival is closely tied to immunocompetence. As discussed above, a decrease in immunocompetence takes place with age, mostly in the T-cells. What effect does this have or should it have on treatment? A middle-aged person who developed pneumonia would have a cough, maybe some chest pain, some fever, perhaps some shortness of breath. This person would go to a doctor, who would hopefully do a number of diagnostic studies. This would include a history and physical examination and certain laboratory studies, including a sputum examination. The physician would stain and culture the sputum to identify the type of bacteria and the antibiotics to which they might be susceptible. He/she would also do a blood count, since an elevated white blood count would also be a sign of bacterial infection. Because in pneumonia there is a significant incidence of bacteremia (bacteria in the blood), the doctor should also take a blood culture. A chest x-ray would presumably show a cloudiness, indicating the infiltrate—the site of pneumonitis or pneumonia. The physician would start the patient on an appropriate antibiotic, and after about 24 to 36 hours the patient would be feeling better. The temperature would have decreased, as would the coughing and the chest pain. The patient would then have what has been called a "walking pneumonia." The physician, however, would keep the patient on the antibiotic for 7 to 10 days, and have the patient come back for a checkup. At this time the physician would preferably supplement the physical examination with another x-ray, which would probably show virtually complete resolution of the pneumonia. There might be a little shadow, a little soft infiltrate left, but the physician would not worry about that. The physician would stop the antibiotic, and the patient would be fine. The physician would have the patient return in another week or two for another check; perhaps he/she would take another x-ray to show complete resolution of the pneumonia. At this time the radiographic shadow would be completely gone.

An 80-year-old who developed pneumonia would hopefully receive at least as careful an examination. The doctor would take an electrocardiogram (ECG), because there are frequently cardiac complications in pneumonia, especially in older people. The doctor would identify the infecting organism by sputum smear, culture and sensitivities; do blood counts, blood cultures, and other indicated tests; and start the patient on the appropriate antibiotic.

Unfortunately, it is often the case that older people frequently get fewer diagnostic studies. There is a tendency not to look as carefully, or to do as much evaluation of older people.

Instead of feeling better within 24 to 36 hours after institution of antibiotics, the 80-year-old person may not feel much better until 48 to 72 hours have elapsed. The doctor would keep up the antibiotic, usually for the same amount of time as for a younger person (7 to 10 days), and then have the patient return for follow-up; at that time, the physician would check the chest and take another x-ray, which would show virtually complete resolution of pneumonia—perhaps just a slight shadow remaining. The doctor would stop the antibiotic, and the patient would be fine for a day.

If the patient were in a nursing home, the caring situation might be the same. For some reason, however, antibiotics frequently seem to be stopped on Friday night in nursing homes. The patient is fine on Saturday, but on Sunday morning, the nurses notice that the patient has a little temperature, maybe 100° F (37.8°C). The patient does not eat as well, and the staff says, "Well, we'll wait to see how the patient is tomorrow. The doctor's away golfing today, or he's at the lake for the weekend, and it's hard to get hold of him." When Monday morning arrives, the patient is moribund. He/she may be comatose, in shock, and virtually at death's door.

What has happened? The older person had that little bit of residual infiltrate at the end of the antibiotic treatment. It takes approximately a day after discontinuation for the drug to be excreted or metabolized, or both. Then, without the residual antibiotic in the system, the older person's decreased immunocompetence isn't sufficient to bring about resolution of that little bit of residual pneumonia. What happens is that when the antibiotic is eliminated, the pneumonia reactivates, spreads, and becomes lethal.

In other words, the decreased immunocompetence of the older person requires different and more assiduous treatment and follow-up. This same problem is seen not only in pneumonia, but in urinary tract infections; it is seen in septicemia, bloodstream infections, and infections in all parts of the body. The special problems presented by health care management of older people are largely unrecognized.

It is still unclear how long the older person needs treatment. Some older people appear to have fairly good immunocompetence and may do as well with the standard antibiotic treatment. Some may require considerably longer. The judgment has to be based on the clinical findings: Older people generally should be treated until there is complete resolution of infection, because they may be immunologically compromised.

These are only some examples of the different physiology of older persons, which call for different treatment. It is important that nurses and allied health professionals know this, as well as physicians; and that people in general be aware of the kinds of attention and care that older people need.

CURRENT UNITED STATES POLICY ON HEALTH CARE FOR THE ELDERLY

The general approach of our country to the care and treatment of older persons bears mentioning, particularly those areas in which we should exercise some caution, from a philosophic point of view. When the federal government set up the Medicare program, the provision was included that older persons in nursing homes had to be seen at least once a month by their physician to provide a bare minimum of attendance. This was considered laudable, as that would at least provide one visit; the intent was to provide a stimulus to encourage visitations and evaluation by physicians. However, when fiscal constraints became the determinants of federal Medicare policy, there was a very interesting change in that regulation. It now reads that Medicare will not cover more than one visit per month. What originated as a limitation on the minimum number, has now been perverted into a limitation on the maximum. A very interesting change.

Much attention is given to the increased cost of medical care, and the federal government and others are saying that we have to hold the costs down. We are told that we are spending 8% and 9% of our national income on health care, so we have to do something about it by decreasing the amount spent on health care.

Who is to say what is the proper amount to spend? The proper amount is, no doubt, between zero and 100% of the national income, but it has yet to be determined that 9% is too much. No one appreciates waste: Unprofessionally indicated procedures, tests, and overutilization are undesirable, but equally undesirable are underutilization and arbitrary fiscal constraints on the health and well-being of people. The federal government can spend 25% of our national budget for what is loosely termed defense; is 8% to 9% of our national product too much to spend for health care? It is a moot point. Before one can say that it is too much, one needs to know what would be considered optimal care, and what it would cost. The reason for such concern is predicated upon the fear of where the squeeze will be applied; that is, where the low priority for health care delivery will be placed. Will it be put on the people who are no longer "economically productive" in our country?

Last summer a new agency was established in Washington, D.C. Called the Health Care Financing Administration, it is a division of HEW, and it is responsible for Medicare, Medicaid, and the Professional Standards Review Organization (PSRO), the so-called peer review of physician performance. In an internal memorandum transmitted by the director of the Health Care Financing Administration to the secretary of HEW for use at a meeting with the president of the United States, there were some very interesting proposals.[1]

For example, one of the statements was that the cost of caring for an "unwanted" child's medical expenses in the first year of life is about $1,000 a year more than the cost of an abortion. Therefore, as a cost-saving initiative, the federal government should encourage the performance of abortion of "unwanted" children because the savings would amount to about $1 billion a year.

Another recommendation was even more fascinating: It pointed out that more than 20% of the health care costs of Medicare are incurred by people in their last year of life. This is probably true. The recommendation was that the federal government encourage the adoption of living wills, because it would result in an estimated savings of $1.2 billion a year. Such savings would result if only one out of every four older persons had a living will, which would preclude medical care in the last year of life of that person.

In this day of priorities we have to be very careful about who sets up the priorities, and how they are implemented. The people who perhaps have the least voice, or who are the least able to have a voice in priority setting, will be the older persons.

We have to base our health care policy decisions on more humanistic and more rational means, and not on the basis of what fiscal administrators and cost accountants decide.

Why do we have to do it now? Why do we have to think about how older people are being treated now, and how they will be treated in the future? Because the systems and institutions that we develop now for older persons are those in which we ourselves will live and die.

REFERENCE

1.   Reiff, T. R. It can happen here. *Journal of the American Medical Association, 239*(26), 2761–2762, 1978.

PHARMACOLOGY OF AGING
Eric Pfeiffer

Greater emphasis needs to be placed, not on misuse, abuse, or nonuse (i.e., underutilization), but on the appropriate use of drugs on and by elderly persons. Some distinctions must be drawn among misuse, abuse, and nonuse. The word misuse might most appropriately be applied to the inadvertent adverse effects that result from the prescribing, giving, and taking of medication. Abuse has referred to the voluntary overuse of medication largely for hedonistic reasons, while nonuse is probably the biggest medication problem of all, involving either inappropriate doses or inappropriate levels or lengths of time.

From this author's point of view as a behavioral scientist, the focus here will be upon five kinds of behavior with regard to the pharmacology of aging.

First of all, we must consider the behavior of drugs in the physiological systems of the older person, on, essentially, drug pharmacokinetics. Second, the prescribing behaviors of the two principal prescribers in the United States today will be described—the M.D. and the TV. Our third concern is the issue of dispensing behaviors: i.e., the actions of pharmacists, the changes that have come about, and the resultant effects upon clientele. The older persons themselves and their drug-taking behaviors are a fourth concern; and finally, we must discuss drug-pushing behaviors.

THE BEHAVIOR OF DRUGS IN OLDER PERSONS

Drugs behave differently in older people. The extent to which they behave differently varies materially, depending on the nature of the drugs and the specific age of individuals, as well as other factors that are more likely determined by physiological age (i.e., distance from death) than chronological age (i.e., distance from birth).

There is one category of drugs whose behavior in older persons is not vastly different: the antibiotic/antimicrobial agents, which fight infectious disease. But virtually all other drugs require substantial adjustments in dosage because of a variety of age-dependent cumulative factors that affect blood levels, tissue responsivity, and changes in absorption patterns. The fact that many drugs are poorly absorbed by older persons is significant because it leads to lower body levels of drugs, which is an important issue in drug-taking behaviors of older people.

On the other hand, factors tending to increase blood levels are changes in the metabolic process. Enzyme systems do not necessarily break drugs down either to active or inactive components. Drug storage and excretion are to a considerable degree influenced by total body composition: The amount of fat in the body increases with age, while the amount of water decreases. The net result of these factors, however, is usually the requirement of fewer dosages and fewer milligrams to achieve the same therapeutic level or the same serum level. Some distinction must be drawn between these two because we still do not know exactly whether it is serum level, or some other (closer to the actual tissue) kind of level, of drugs that makes the critical difference.

In the brain, for instance, there is a kind of a dropping out of brain cells at a rate of about .8% per year, beginning at about age 25 or 30. When an individual reaches 65 or 70 years of age, the brain tissue has been reduced by 30 or 40%. The person is, in fact, still safe, but he/she is figuratively walking around on the edge of a cliff. That relatively small change in the surrounding environment of the tissue can lead to drastic changes, just as could one step toward the precipice of the cliff.

Very little is known with respect to the regularity with which drugs vary in their behavior. What we know of drugs' behavior is essentially their misbehavior. That is, we have made everyone our experimental subject, to allow us to study basic pharmacokinetics, which are totally uncontrolled.

We can always learn from the misadventures that the old have with drugs. The FDA is designed to test the behavior of single drugs in essentially healthy persons who are about age 25, and who may be suffering from one disease. Older people, however, tend to have three or four diseases; they may be taking three or four medications; and they are certainly not 25! Virtually no basic pharmacokinetic studies have been done on drug behavior in subjects with multiple impairments, taking several drugs. This is an enormously important area for formal scientific investigation. At this point we are allowing older people essentially to serve as a kind of an experimental group to tell us something about how drugs should not be used on the elderly.

The National Institute on Aging (NIA), however, has made the pharmacology of aging a very high priority for new research; it wll be funded if good research protocols are in fact forthcoming. The director of that institute is fully cognizant of the multiplicity of issues.

DRUG-PRESCRIBING BEHAVIORS

Physicians have not been taught in medical schools that drug dosages must be drastically adjusted for older people, both in terms of frequency and in terms of magnitude, in order to be consistent with their physiological changes. They had not been taught when I went to medical school, and they are still not being taught in very many places. A few places are beginning to introduce gerontological content in their curricula, and it appears that a requirement is being included for practical nurses for gerontological content. It might be time to include gerontological content in the curricula of health practitioners in general, not only some segments of it.

The physician who does not know how to prescribe medications for older people is not alone in this picture. Another side to the story that requires illustration is that many patients come to the physician with a complaint, fully expecting that they will walk out with a medication in hand. The pressure to give a prescription is high from the elderly patient population themselves. For example, physicians in family practice at times try to do a lot of psychotherapy themselves; they might call it counseling, or simply talking over problems. They discovered that many patients seen in this more enlightened way—in which they did not use drugs as a substitute for human interaction—would say, "I don't understand, Dr. Stewart, why you charged me for that visit; you didn't do anything. All you did was talk to me."

Thus there is a high level of expectation on the part of many families of older people and of the older people themselves, that one of the things the doctor must do is give some visible evidence for them to take away, that they are, in fact, receiving treatment. There are tremendous pressures on the doctor to prescribe.

Television as Prescriber

One of the most important physicians in this country is, so far as I know, totally unlicensed and very powerful. On the surface it seems to cost nothing to get your prescriptions from the television. The results may be disastrous or inefficient, or at least an expenditure that will do no good. Extensive studies have shown that a change in television advertising has resulted in drastic changes in the pattern of compounds sold at the local drugstore counter. All the same, the unknown factors of age-dependent changes in drug absorption, excretion, metabolic breakdown, and storage, apply to over-the-counter preparations as well as to prescription medications.

Through much of television advertising, there is the implication that drugs will solve problems such as loneliness and the negative feelings often associated with retirement or with many other normative human interactions that might more appropriately be handled through counseling or through social interaction. Thus the pressure is very high to take drugs for various kinds of reasons without any great detailed knowledge of what a drug is and how it behaves.

No patient should take any drug without understanding it. Patients should learn to be assertive and talk back to their doctors if the doctors will not bother to explain what a drug does. The same need exists with respect to their prescribing doctor on television: Unless that doctor talks back to them, they should not take the drugs he prescribes.

DRUG-DISPENSING BEHAVIOR

Pharmacy has changed a lot since it began as a kind of a friendly drugstore operation. The pharmacist was in fact called "Doc" in the old days, and he was used a kind of primary care practitioner. In the present drugstore, such as the Eckerds, or Scaggs, or Rexall chains, you have to walk past a number of other items (rubber gloves, scrub brushes, milk, bread); past the over-the-counter prescriptions counter, where it is hoped you will actually buy some other medication before you get to the pharmacist. When you get to the pharmacist, you find him/her sitting on a high platform behind a little glass wall.

Imagine a little old lady coming up to the platform, reaching up, and handing the prescription to the pharmacist up there. He sort of grunts, and takes it away. There is no place to sit and wait. Now suppose she wanted to ask the pharmacist a question. There is no way of doing it, even if the pharmacist were accessible. If it were a question dealing with a personal health-related matter, such as, "Is constipation a side effect of this medication?", would she want to be asking this while somebody right next to her was picking out a hair coloring agent?

The current pharmacy is essentially a product of orientation service; not a service orientation. In Florida, there has been a practice of discounting the price of pharmaceutical products. This, it would appear, is a very poor practice. The discount should be, if it is going to be given, for the benefit of older people in providing a counseling service about what the medication might do. The new era of clinical pharmacy will have to come to the rescue of these older persons and their physicians in order to change this pattern.

DRUG-TAKING BEHAVIOR

Drug-taking behavior on the part of older persons is very erratic. Recently a drugstore chain in Florida had a contest that illustrates this point. They said, "Throw away all of your medications; they may not be effective anymore." The assumption was that many people were still using medications that were prescribed a long time ago. They had contests as to who could bring in the oldest bottle of medicine, still dated; and it came out 1937.

It is a fact that approximately 80% of drugs prescribed for older people on a certain date are not consumed. They sit on shelves. That means 80% of drugs prescribed (and paid for) are not actually consumed for that purpose at that time. They may be consumed later by the same person, by a family member, or by a friend. The rationale is that since it helped my backache, maybe it will help yours. It may not have been the same kind of backache.

There is a fair amount of trading of drugs and a fair amount of suspicion of drugs. An almost unknown pattern of drug usage exists, including taking more than prescribed, taking substantially less than prescribed, and taking substitute medications purchased over the counter, perhaps through the counsel of television advertisements. It is basically a chaotic picture, and it stems from the fact that the doctor handed the patient three slips of paper to be filled by a pharmacist who filled three bottles, and whose instructions the older person can neither read nor follow.

DRUG ADMINISTRATION

There is no such thing as a standard dosage for older persons. We do not today know what constitutes a standard dosage on any given specific product for an older person, because older persons can respond identically to younger persons in regard to drug dosage, or they may require 75% or 50% or 25% of the usual dosage. That is, virtually every one of any major medication becomes an individual experiment in titration between the physician and his patient. This requires that either the patient, a family member, or a professional staff person be available to monitor both the positive benefits anticipated from the taking of a medication, and the various adverse effects that might be expected to occur; in this way, changes in medication may be made to adjust the drug level to the effective, not the toxic, level.

This has some interesting implications. It means that several things must be known about the patient. First of all, is the patient intellectually capable of reporting such information? We need to know whether or not the older person suffers from memory deficit. The moment one says, take this medication

Principles of Drug Administration with Elderly Patients

1. There is no standard dosage for older persons.
2. Start one drug at a time.
3. Use as few drugs as possible, the fewest number of times a day.
4. Ascertain whether or not the patient is taking a medication for the same condition for which he/she comes to the physician.
5. The patient, a family member, or a health care professional must monitor both positive and adverse effects of the drug.
6. There must be a regular drug review.
7. Make the older person your fulltime partner through detailed instruction and explanation.
8. The same medication may have different effects upon the person as he/she grows older.

---

four times a day, or take it with meals, etc., an intellectual demand is being made that cannot be met by the 15% of older people who have significant memory deficit. A simple test of intellectual functioning must be made on the older person who comes to the physician's office alone. The clinician also must inquire who else might be available in case the person does in fact have significant memory deficit. Somebody else should observe the patient and report upon changes in symptoms or the occurrence of side effects.

Never assume that the patient is not already taking a medication for the same condition for which he/she comes to the physician. Frequently patients come to the doctor and present a set of symptoms, but will not say specifically, spontaneously at least, that they are already taking digitalis, or an antihypertensive agent, or an antianxiety agent, for the same exact condition for which they are now coming to the physician. They are simply not satisfied with the results.

The importance of starting with a clean slate cannot be overemphasized. Prescribing for older persons is a major undertaking, not to be done lightly. The best way of starting with a clean slate is to say, "Bring your tired, your poor bottles of medicine; bring them all in a plastic bag, and we'll look at them, and we'll probably throw them out." This is certainly a good way to find out what the patient has been taking, and it is also a good way to get an idea of the medical history of the patient. So it is best to get the patient or his family member to bring in all medications before prescribing new ones.

Start one drug at a time. The only exception to this would be if the patient is in a hospital setting where the physician can effectively control and supervise drug taking, or where he/she has established a pattern of multiple drug use. But even that is risky without day-to-day observations of symptomatology, blood pressure, laboratory findings, and so on. With very rare exceptions, such as the treatment of acute pulmonary edema, it is critical that all of the medications we pour into the system at one time be observed for effects, both positive and negative.

The continuance of medication may need to be for substantially longer periods of time than in younger persons, especially in the areas of antibiotics. This is actually a general principle in regard to aging patients. Elderly persons are quite responsive to treatments, but the treatment must often be modified, and one of the ways it must be modified is in term of length of treatment. This is particularly true of antibiotics for infectious diseases.

This is also true, just by way of an extension of general principle, for the treatment of, say, congestive failure, or recovery from a myocardial infarction or recovery from stroke. Because if we follow the PSRO model of saying thirteen days for a coronary for a 45 year old person, we'll give an extra two days for the older patient. Otherwise, we will quit treating that patient before he's well, and he may be permanently disabled. If we say it might take four weeks to give physical therapy and speech therapy to a young person with a stroke or a hemorrage in the brain, it might take twice, or two and a half times that long, in order to effectively lead to the rehabilitation of an older person. If we quit too soon, we will quit before we have had an opportunity to lead to recovery from illness.

There's another side to this issue of time, however, which is related to the prescribing of medication. One cannot make the assumption that the patient will continue to require medication forever, even for some of the chronic diseases. This is particularly true in disease entities such as hypertension, where after a period of treatment of three months or six months or even a year, often times discontinuation of medication is possible without significant return of hypertension. Hypertension can be controlled on substantially lower dosages than was previously thought possible. The same is true for diabetes, and to a lesser degree of congestive heart failure.

The basic point is that there must be a regular drug review, rather than a regular drug renewal. Too often the requirements for a review of drugs have simply been requirements for signing the doctor's name to something already written by someone else, because there has not been any sensitive review of this issue.

This raises the same point that is raised by the much-discussed topic of drug holidays. Drug holidays, by the way, are not a day in which one takes a lot of drugs; rather, the notion refers to the simple element of drug review, and generally reduced dosages.

To illustrate, a Dr. Brown, who lives in Providence, Rhode Island, was a remarkable, rather stout lady of about 65 when she had this experience. (She is probably in her early 70s now.) She went to see her doctor one day, and he said, "Oh, Dr. Brown, you have high blood pressure, and I'll have to put you on some medication." He put her on some antihypertensive medication, and told her that should take care of her. She took it for 3 days; on the third day, whenever she tried to get up, she fell down. She went back to the doctor, and when the doctor measured her blood pressure, it dropped fully 70 points from her sitting position to her standing position. She felt faint and dizzy. The doctor became alarmed, and decided to quit giving her the medication, and she went home. Dr. Brown is not a timid lady by any means, but she did not once talk back to her doctor. She sat at home in her apartment in Providence, and she thought, "Well, gee whiz, if the medicine was supposed to do me good in the first place, you know, it's too bad I can't take it any more. On the other hand, if it did me harm, I guess I shouldn't be taking it anymore. Maybe what I'll do is take it every other day." Without consulting her doctor, she made that choice, and her blood pressure was very well controlled.

This illustration demonstrates that we are learning that older people themselves really have had to be the guinea pigs to figure out what to do, because we have lacked the scientific information to provide them. We have had to learn from older people what to do with regard to prescribing and drug-taking behaviors. So drug holidays have nothing magical about them; we are just dealing with another basic principle. The very lowest dosage is used that produces the required therapeutic effect; and given the fact that excretion and metabolic breakdown are far slower, it turns out that there is a hidden benefit in this system. Once-daily dosage is often sufficient, rather than several times daily.

Another principle to bear in mind, in order to get correct drug dosage, is to make it as simple as it can possibly be. An interesting memory device has been produced in Germany, which is supposed to simplify things. It shows the 7 days of the week across the top, and four drug dosages; it just assumes that everybody would be taking qid medications, and that the different qid medications would be packaged into this device at different times of the day. Even an individual who is relatively intact intellectually would get very confused trying to use such a device. Actually, the best memory device is to use the fewest drugs possible, the fewest number of times a day. Memory devices, however, do have a real role to play. To our young women on birth control pills we have not hesitated to give memory devices that say they should take one pill a day for 21 days; they can tell when they have taken it and then they are off the pill for the 7 days. We have not yet developed this as a systematic form of memory device available to older people, and we must work on this issue as well.

A point already alluded to in regard to principles of drug-prescribing behavior is that wherever possible, except when there is serious intellectual deficit, you should make the older person your full-time partner in the giving of medication. That is, you should teach older persons exactly, and in detail, why it is they are taking a certain medication, what that medication does, what the risks of that medication are, and how that might change over a period of time.

It is important to remember that the same medication prescribed for older persons may have different effects as they grow yet older, and even lower dosages may be required because further physiological changes have taken place.

A very dramatic illustration of how the same drug taken regularly over a period of years changes its efficacy and impact and clout (positively and negatively, as one may wish to consider it) is the use of alcohol. The healthy normal adult who has, say, two martinis with dinner every day will essentially be drinking four martinis when he reaches 65 or 70. There is clear-cut evidence that alcohol is handled by the aging body in substantially different ways. As older persons continue lifelong habits of alcohol ingestion, their responses to it may be sudden blackouts, inability to perform sexually, memory deficit the morning after the drinking event, and other side effects that are essentially the result of having a differential impact from the same dosage, if you will, that they have taken for years.

Indications for Specific Drugs

In every aspect of the field of aging, even though persons are not prescribing medications, it is useful to have some general understanding of the purposes, actions, and side effects of some of these medications. A considerable amount of attention will be given in this discussion to psychotropic drugs, with a lesser emphasis upon the various cardiovascular drugs, as well as some mention of the analgesic, pain-killer, antiinflammatory drugs.

The psychotropic drugs are not only still the most frequently used drugs; they are frequently used for the wrong indications. This is one of the basic principles in prescribing in general, but is particularly important with respect to psychotropic drugs. Drugs are not a substitute for people.

Many drugs are utilized as substitutes for people, that is, for human interaction, for counseling, for psychotherapy, for crisis intervention, for friendship, and to combat social isolation. For that reason, one must stress the real indications for which drugs are to be used, and, in general, use them as an adjunct to a therapeutic relationship, and not as a substitute at all.

Four or five major categories of psychotropic drugs must be understood, because approximately 20% to 25% of elderly patients are on some type of psychotropic medication. This is the proportion of people living in the community. The proportion in long-term care facilities who are on psychotropic medications is probably closer to 50%, or even 70% or 80%.

Psychotropic drugs are psychologically active drugs that influence people's behavior or the way they feel. They include antidepressants, major tranquilizers, minor tranquilizers, sedatives, stimulants; and also some unclassified drugs that supposedly affect behavior including vitamins E and B_{15}.

Antidepressants

The principal category to be addressed is the antidepressant drugs. Some of the most well-known are: imipramine (Tofranil), desipramine (Norpramin, Pertofrane), doxepin (Sinequan), and amitriptyline (Elavil). There are a few others. There are always new drug companies coming along with "me too" drugs that are essentially the same chemical. They are largely tricyclic antidepressants, but some monoamine oxidase (MAO) inhibitors fit into this category also. Their indications should not be a temporary feeling of sadness, or being upset or anxious, or distrustful; rather, they should be the clinical occurrence of a depressive syndrome. This includes the presence of psychological sadness; loss of interest, which continues over a period of weeks and months; and the presence of physical signs of depression, such as loss of appetite, loss of weight, and sleeplessness. The continued existence of these symptoms is an indication for antidepressant drugs in conjunction with psychotherapeutic efforts.

The antidepressants, as a class of drugs, produce three major kinds of side effects. One is that in about 1% to 4% of people they cause a delirium that resembles acute schizophrenia and can result in total disorientation. This often leads to an acute psychiatric admission, and a previously well-behaved elderly woman may compensate and talk and swear, and may have hallucinations, largely visual, but some auditory as well. Psychiatric residents will sometimes misdiagnose these as acute schizophrenic reactions, which probably do not occur at all in older persons. Rather, they are delirious reactions in response to some of the antidepressant drugs prescribed in normal adult dosages, and they are less likely to occur if dosages are kept lower than the normal adult dosage of approximately 200 or 300 mg/day.

A second category of side effects is in the cardiovascular area, where a number of things can go wrong: arrhythmias (irregular heartbeats), orthostatic hypotension (i.e., a tendency to black out and fall down upon beginning to get up), and occasionally, sudden hypertension.

The third category of symptoms applies primarily to men, and it affects the genitourinary system. A frequent illness in older men is benign prostatic hypertrophy (BPH), which can lead to urinary shutdown; male patients may also experience dysphoric reactions accompanying sexual intercourse, varying with individuals. They may experience loss of libido or be unable to reach ejaculation when on the drugs; some otherwise uncomfortable feelings also occur, which are hard to classify but are among the major side effects. A decision must be made whether the side effects are worth the possible improvements in this regard. Adjustments in dosage may help, but these are very serious side effects. In the *Physician's Desk Reference* (*PDR*), the number of side effects listed for the antidepressants is among the longest of any kind of medication in the entire armamentarium of the pharmaceutical industry. Yet they are effective in bringing about recovery from the depression that may lead to suicide if not treated. They should not be utilized for minor declines, as when something goes wrong during the day, but only for serious depressive illness, and then they should be closely supervised.

The three kinds of side effects described above should be shared with patients in order to get adequate feedback from them. At the same time, regular assessments should help determine whether some improvements are beginning to occur. On occasion, it may be well to admit patients to the hospital for 2 or 3 days, in order to start them on antidepressant drugs. Although improvements with antidepressant medication do not occur until about 2 or 3 weeks after initiation of therapy, the side effects occur almost immediately. Thus, the importance of closer monitoring of the starting dosage of antidepressant medication cannot be overemphasized.

Major Tranquilizers

The most commonly used major tranquilizers are chlorpromazine (Thorazine), thioridazine (Mellaril), trifluoperazine (Stelazine), and haloperidol (Haldol). There are some new ones, but they have not come into as much usage. In younger people the major tranquilizers are used as antipsychotic agents particularly in schizophrenic reactions, sometimes in rather large dosages. Their indication in the older person is paranoia. Paranoia in older persons should not be interpreted as the kind of serious mental illness that it is in younger people. Older people often become frightened because they have to fill in the blank spaces about what is going on in their environment, and they cannot hear as well; they often have to make up what they are saying. When they don't remember, they may say, "Gari, why did you steal my watch? I can't find it; what did you do with it?" By the time she finishes speaking, the patient may not even know who she is. There may be a caretaker, a daughter, or a nurse in the home who is very much offended at being accused of stealing from this "paranoid" patient. But she is not really paranoid; she just cannot figure out where she put her watch anymore. Since there is a stranger in the house, that person must have stolen it. The problem with this is that it alienates a lot of people; a patient may even lose a caretaker in the process. Such paranoid symptomatology, which is fraught by fear and misunderstanding, can sometimes be very effectively treated by low dosages of the major tranquilizers. Occasionally, as an adjunct to severe agitation, the major tranquilizers may also be used. Dosages here probably range from 25% to 30% of a normal adult dosage.

A few additional points need to be mentioned by way of general information about how to use these agents. They are probably best given once a day, at bedtime, because they tend to make people a little sleepy. These drugs tend to have their antiparanoid effects throughout the day, even if they are given at night, and the drowsiness will not occur in the daytime. Generally, such a dosage is quite sufficient.

Minor Tranquilizers

Next we consider the minor tranquilizers, their legitimate indications, and some of the problems that result with their usage. The minor tranquilizers include the big sellers in the industry. The number one and three drugs as of the most recent readings are diazepam (Valium) and chlordiazepoxide (Librium). Other minor tranquilizers include such drugs as meprobamate (Miltown) and the barbiturates, and generally, the class of sedatives. Alcohol is also in the same category, although it is not available through the same channels or the same outlets, except in certain states where liquor can be purchased at the drugstore.

The indications for minor tranquilizers are acute anxiety states such as occur in older people who run into adverse life situations that they cannot handle, leading them into uncontrolled panic and anxiety states. When these medications are used for a period of 3 or 4 days, they will reduce the anxiety physiologically, enough so that the person can now cope with the situation. They are useful in short-term crisis situations, either as daytime sedatives or as nighttime hypnotics.

People may become very upset over adverse events, such as being told that they have to move from their home and be admitted to a nursing home. No amount of talking will help in some of these instances, and the use of a minor tranquilizer then is highly indicated; it will control the anxiety so that soon the patient can begin to cope with the situation and take real-life corrective measures. All too frequently, however, such occasions initiate long-term use of these agents; herein lies the problem, since these agents tend to require higher dosages in order to produce the same effects after a period of perhaps a week or 10 days. They pose the same problems as do other medications in that they are slowly excreted.

Anybody of age 75 or so who is taking 5 mg of Valium four times a day is going to walk around with a buzz on all the time. Now that wouldn't be so bad in itself it it were just a mental buzz, but it may affect the person's entire physiological system. Many hip fractures leading to death are in fact caused by the injurious use or the continuation of these medications. Sometimes this occurs when patients themselves increase their drug dosages. Sometimes irregularity of dosage leads to elevated blood levels in the older person and the resulting higher responsivity in terms of equilibrium components. Falls are very, very common among older persons on these medications, not to mention the drug-induced intellectual and memory decline that may also occur.

One other unfortunate occurrence is related to the sudden cessation of use of minor tranquilizing drugs. For instance, someone may be taking them regularly, and upon admission to a hospital for a hernia operation or for some minor matter, may not mention this fact. Thus the intern or doctor will not prescribe continuation of the medication. After 2 or 3 days the person may go into drug withdrawal and have convulsions and delirium.

Minor tranquilizers are indicated for short-term use and not over the long run, with only one possible exception: that of sleep patterns and sleep disturbances. A lot of older people have problems with sleep, sometimes as a result of illness or other physical disturbances. Pain such as that associated with arthritis may keep the person awake. Other sleep problems are the result of psychiatric illnesses; namely, acute anxiety episodes or serious depression. The most common of all these changes in sleep patterns are normative, which neither the older person himself nor those around him may recognize as such.

We all know that the sleep pattern of babies is totally different from that of adults. We did not recognize until very recently that older people have a different sleep pattern from younger people or young adults. It is characterized by very little deep sleep; three to four irregular awakenings at night, but no difficulty in going back to sleep. If provision is made for a lighted hallway and access to the refrigerator and the bathroom (which is where most people go when they wake up at night), the problems are over.

In addition, the older person naps for about half an hour to an hour, two or three times during the day. Thus the sleep pattern is completely changed in the older person. And too often we have observed a nurse in a long-term care facility shaking Miss Jones, saying, "Don't go to sleep now, you won't be able to sleep at night." Further, they insist that Miss Jones stay asleep for 8 hours at night, administering a sleeping medication to help.

Sedatives and Stimulants

There apparently are some differences among sleeping medications of the sedative variety. Some practitioners think that barbiturates are particularly bad, as there are idiosyncratic reactions to barbiturates. Nonetheless, many patients do perfectly well with barbiturates, and they are not necessarily off limits. However, there are plenty of alternatives available. No sleeping medication in this category of drugs, such as barbiturate or chloral hydrate, has any effect on the sleep pattern at all if given 14 days in a row or longer. What they don't lose their effectiveness in, is in clouding morning consciousness. As they hang over until the morning, they may cause some impairment in memory function for either the whole day or at least a portion of the day after administration.

Some recent work indicates that the benzodiazepines, especially Valium in a dosage of about 5 mg, at any bedtime may be among the safest of sleep-inducing agents that can be given, for two reasons: (1) it seems less likely to lose effectiveness over a period of time; (2) it cannot very easily be used as a suicidal agent. Relatively few people have died from overdosages of Valium, and those who have, have taken them with large combinations of alcohol, rather than Valium alone. Many people have died from barbiturate overdosage, however: They just cannot get to sleep despite the barbiturate, so they take the whole bottle, often dying as a result.

Alcohol is the most frequently used psychotropic agent. It is probably used by 90% of old people, and by 97% of the total adult population. We now know some important things about the use of alcohol; for instance, there are limits to its use. Abstinence is probably a virtue, but not a great virtue. The longevity statistics actually indicate that light to moderate alcohol users tend to live a little longer than people who abstain altogether from alcohol. That is no reason to switch from abstinence to alcohol, because the risk of developing alcoholism is considerable.

Up to about 55 or 60, up to 4 ounces of liquor (not alcohol) per day is probably all right, extended over the full day and not taken all in one sitting. Beyond that amount, there is clear-cut evidence that it reduces life expectancy. Thus there is a kind of curve indicating that nothing is quite as good as having an occasional drink, maybe a glass of wine every day; but when one begins to exceed about 4 ounces, one enters the danger territory. This holds for the entire adult age group.

For the older age group, the dosage needs to be cut in half in order to play safe. There is a negative impact that can affect the myocardium, the liver, the digestive system, the rate of accidents, the suicide rate, among other things. The real alcoholic (about 10% of all drinkers) has a life expectancy 10 years less than that of the average American.

Caffeine has no proven negative effect, except possibly that if some people drink coffee very late at night, they then take sleeping medication in order to go to sleep. The coffee itself is not harmful, but the taking of the sleeping medication may present a problem. Coffee drinking, other than causing sleeplessness or jitteriness, has no proven effect on life expectancy.

There is no level at which nicotine is beneficial; giving up smoking at any age will lead to additional longevity.

Some mention must also be made of the vasodilators, such as Hydergine. They are intended to dilate stenosed arteries in the brain so that better mental functioning can occur. The problem is that in a stenotic artery, the muscles you are trying to relax in the arterial wall have been lined with calcium, and calcium is very hard to relax.

New studies in progress are attempting to determine whether there may be some value in their use, but the evidence thus far is very slim. They produce few if any side effects. It would be difficult to predict which person with some memory deficit will respond positively to these agents. Persons following the principle, "Well, we might as well try it; if there is any chance of doing good, we want to do it," might be well advised to try it for about 3 months. If there are no improvements in the patient's behavior in measurable terms, then there is probably no reason to continue the medication.

Hydergine is a particularly interesting drug that nobody understands, although it is highly promoted. It has at times been used as an antidepressant agent or as a memory-improving agent, and most recently has been called an agent for curing the "soft symptoms" of senility. Although it is unclear what the soft symptoms of senility are, such statements are based on repeated controlled studies indicating that certain kinds of behaviors (i.e., manner of dressing, amount of interaction with peers, some mood changes) seem to improve in about 15% of older people who are given this drug. It would be difficult to predict that 15 out of 100 will have these soft positive changes, but the results are statistically significant. There are no significant side effects from Hydergine, but continued use for more than 3 months or so without demonstrable effects would be a waste of money.

A disorder called hypochondriasis often appears in older people, somewhat more often in women than men: This is excessive bodily concern, on the assumption that one has a physical disease, even when a doctor cannot find much that is wrong. These people are focusing on their body's functioning because their social functioning has become empty and unsatisfying. They will hear their heart beating in the night, just as most people do. They will look at their muscles, and see a muscle twitch. They will hear borborygmi (stomach growling); or feel their heart skip a beat occasionally and a kind of twinge (a common experience for most people); and say that something is wrong. Something is wrong: Life is not as pleasing as it once was.

These patients are sick and in need of care, and they often have been to many doctors before (not often to psychiatrists). In such instances, there are some things not to do. One should neither tell the patient that there is nothing wrong with him, nor do extensive diagnostic workups (which are a temptation) because everything else has been tried. Doctors sometimes get so impatient that they will perform some uncomfortable procedures such as a proctoscopy.

What does help is accepting the patient as someone who is sick and in need of care. One of the ways of doing that and conveying that is to give the patient regular but infrequent appointments. Such patients should never be put on a prn status (call me when you need me); for that time is always right now. A regular appointment should be made for a certain time and place. The date can be quite far off, but it has to be fixed.

Another useful "treatment" in hypochondriasis is placebo medication, which is essentially either inert or in very low dosages. Since it has either no or very slight side effects, it is very useful. A symbolic connection is established between the doctor and the patient. The bottle displays the patient's and a doctor's name; and it has a big Rx linking the two together. That is a powerful connection, saying to the outside world that this patient is under doctor so-and-so's care.

Some of these patients are mildly depressed; some of them are mildly anxious. The use of very low dosages of any of the antianxiety agents is probably as good a placebo as any, although some pharmacies carry wonderfully colored placebos that are totally inert.

Food as a drug should be addressed, however briefly. Food is used by many people as a drug; that is, as a substitute for people. It is probably one of the major unaddressed health problems with which individual physicians have not adequately dealt. Some physicians have done very well with the problem, but the failure rate (that is, the return to overweight conditions) has been very high. Overeating is an unsolved health hazard that has to be addressed by a public health approach: essentially this means through media education that is informed by physician input, rather than on a one-to-one basis. (See also Chapter 10 on this subject.)

Chapter 3

GERIATRIC PSYCHIATRY: PHYSICIAN–PATIENT GOALS IN THE MENTAL HEALTH OF OLD PEOPLE

Alex Comfort

It is to the physician, not the psychiatrist, that the old and their relatives turn for crisis intervention. This is fitting, for at no period of life are mental and physical symptoms more closely interlinked. The physician who treats old patients must either address their mental problems, at least by understanding their relation to nonpsychiatric medication, or run the risk of being himself actively nosogenic. It is, moreover, the physician who by careful physical examination can save the old from psychiatric institutional commitment and restore them to worthwhile living, an immensely satisfying exercise when it works. Thus much of geriatric psychiatry is part of the normal equipment of all who see patients over the age of 65.

Old people suffer from the psychiatric problems common to the human condition. They also suffer from psychiatric problems peculiar to age, and peculiar to age in our culture. Peculiar to age is the tendency for physical diseases that earlier in life present sharply and specifically, to present in geriatric practice in a muted or nonspecific form. Typical syndromes are blurred:

Coronary heart disease, pneumonia, urinary infection, thyro-toxicosis, and many other medical conditions may be stripped of their usual signatures and appear as a nonspecific combination of mental and physical symptoms such as withdrawal, mental blunting, loss of mobility, and physical weakness. This syndrome, popularly called "senility," represents the Shake-spearean "last act." Thus far from being a diagnosis, senility is the geriatric equivalent of failure to thrive in infants.[1] Moreover, mental failure may be the sole presenting symptom of a wide range of pathologies in the old, many of them remediable, and some of them iatrogenic. Of all old people who present with a "psychiatric" problem, between 10% and 30%, according to age, owe their illness to an undiagnosed medical condition, or to the effects of medication, or both. The older the patient, the more often are psychiatric disorders symptomatic, and the first stop must be with the geriatric physician. Geriatric psychiatry is largely medicine, but all good geriatric medicine involves mental health.

Peculiar to aging in our culture is its unique rejection of the old; their exclusion from work and their accustomed social space; their premature burial by society as unpeople; and a rich and erroneous folklore of mental decline, infirmity, asexuality, ineducability, and the normality of causeless mental disorder. Since this folklore is shared by both the old themselves and, unfortunately, also physicians, mental ill health, as well as physical, is seen as requiring no explanation provided the subject is "old." At the same time, the rejecting attitude of our society, and fear of being adjudged senile, forms a ground-base to every theme of mental illness in old age, and must constantly be addressed by a corrective psychotherapy designed to restore self-esteem. This need often be no more than contact with a physician who does not project dislike or contempt for old people.

Geriatric psychiatry is best introduced to students—who need prophylactic injections against the notion that aging involves imbecility and that geriatric medicine is uninteresting and useless—by a series of aphorisms. The first is that *older people are responsive to treatment.* Not only are many apparent psychiatric disorders symptomatic, but they are every bit as treatable in older people as they are in the young, and the same methods are appropriate. The second aphorism is that *old people are not usually sick or crazy:* In fact 75% of persons over 65 describe themselves as "well," and Arthur Rubinstein at 90 is a more representative picture of "normal" age than a sufferer from organic brain disease. Old people who become crazy do so because they always were crazy, because they are sick, or because we drive them crazy.

Major primary psychosis rarely makes its first unheralded appearance in old age: Depression may do so, but schizophrenia virtually never, if we except the "late paraphrenia" occurring in patients with a lifetime of odd beliefs.

As for sickness, it is characteristic of age that disorientation and confusion are relatively easily induced by infection, toxicity, electrolyte changes, and other physical causes, as are convulsions in infants.

As to the idea that we drive them crazy, social ostracism apart, the commonest cause of sudden unexplained mental illness in the old is medication: self-administered, doctor administered, or borrowed from neighbors. Accordingly the first psychodiagnostic step is the withdrawal of all medication that is not life-sustaining, and a thorough review of medication that is. The "plastic bag test"—that is, providing the patient with a bag into which all medication without exception is to be placed may yield tens or even scores of preparations. As a corollary, the student must be aware that in view of the increased homeostatic instability of age, the prescription of *any* drug in old age is no light matter. For the old, there is no such thing as a minor tranquilizer. Neurological and biochemical reserves are reduced; multiple pathology may be present; iatrogenic disease of all kinds, and especially psychiatric, can be precipitated by modest doses of many agents; and falls due to hypotension, ataxia, or confusion can cause the patient's death.

Lastly among aphorisms, *chronic brain syndrome is neither an inevitable concomitant of age, if one lives long enough, nor is it the commonest major psychiatric disorder.*

The commonest truly psychiatric disorder in age is depression. Not only is age in our culture depressing, but there is a basic neuroendocrine shift with aging in the direction characteristic of affective disorder.[2] Depression may be reactive or endogenous; it can be agitated and suicidal; but far more commonly, and more commonly than in the young, it can be confined to somatic equivalents: backache, fatigue, cancer phobia. It can also present as pseudodementia or confusion.

Depression in the old is commonly undiagnosed. It is the most likely basis for sudden or gradual downhill change once sickness and medication are excluded, and it is a medical emergency, both because of the high risk of suicide or death from "giving up," and because it is treatable, often with spectacular benefit. Even when some underlying brain damage exists, lightening of depression can restore social function. When an old person withdraws into self-neglect and isolation, this is far more commonly the result of endogenous depression than the cause of reactive depression. Bereavement, which increases in frequency with age to cover friends and peers as well as spouses, can determine its onset, though grief and sorrow are not diseases and should not be medicated.

According to Linn, "late-life depressions deserve the most serious and even heroic therapeutic efforts, regardless of the age of the patient."[3] Many respond to tricyclic agents, but the dose schedule must be initially homeopathic, since delirium or acute retention are easily induced in the old. One-third of the adult maintenance dosages of amitriptyline or doxepin are typically effective. They should be given at night in a single bolus in order that side effects may be covered by sleep. Early waking is diagnostic of depression in the old, but the temptation to supplement sedative tricyclics with sedatives should be resisted except on a very short-term basis. In unresponsive depression, monoamine oxidase (MAO) inhibitors, or (where distress is acute) electroconvulsive therapy (ECT) should be used: Unilateral ECT to the nondominant hemisphere minimizes postictal confusion in the already confused.[4]

Mania in old age is commonly not expansive but hostile and mixed with depressive elements; it is accordingly often missed, on the mistaken assumption that the old person is senile and is being obnoxious. It is controllable by phenothiazines and other psychotropic agents administered with the caution that applies to all drugs in age, and preventable by lithium[5] with strict laboratory control, since in the old, blood ion levels can fluctuate widely and suddenly. The diazepam group of drugs should be avoided because of the ease with which they induce confusion. Paraldehyde, nasty as it is, has uses in acute mania dependent on the lack of temptation to continue it prophylactically. While mania may be mistaken for senility plus ill temper, alcoholic and drug withdrawal can be mistaken for mania; they commonly surface on admission to hospital. Old people are not only more sensitive to drugs; they more easily become dependent on them.

After depression, the second commonest mental problem of the old, especially in general practice, is probably hypochondriasis, at least as far as physician time is concerned. Underlying depression must first be excluded, if need be by a therapeutic trial. After that, students are enjoined to observe three negatives and four positives.

The negatives are: (1) Do not try to explain to patients the nature of psychosomatic illness; they will go elsewhere. (2) Do not conduct exploratory—and still less, punitive—surgery, proctoscopy, and the like. (3) Do not refer the patient.

The four positives are: (1) Investigate adequately but not obsessionally. (2) Agree that the patient is sick and requires treatment. (3) Then give a placebo; for this purpose an active material such as a tranquilizer should not be used. The traditional "bottle of medicine" possessing trifling activity served the patient as a transitional object and a certificate of permission to be sick, bearing the doctor's name, exhibitable to relatives, and serving as his surrogate to occupy the "interval of therapeutic inactivity." (4) Schedule a definite further appointment. From that point the therapeutic ingredient is time, devoted to establishing confidence and uncovering personal and situational frustrations against which the symptoms are an appeal for help. In psychotherapy with the old, the tyro and even the experienced therapist, who are accustomed to accepting the transference role of parent, may be disconcerted by reversal or rapid alternation in which they find themselves the vehicle of emotions directed not to parents but to children. They may need to remodel their technique and re-examine their countertransferences, often without warning.

ODD BEHAVIOR

It is important to recognize that behavior that is odd in the young is interpreted as "senility" in the old, by common consent of the culture. The young man who assaults little girls is seen as psychopathic; the old man who does so, even when his access to more normal sexual gratification is restricted by opportunity or by infirmity, is described as "senile."

Persons whose behavior was odd in youth may become odder with age as the pressure of societal rejection comes to bear on them. Paranoia at any age is cover for unexplainable experiences. In the old these may include the attempt to cover sensory losses such as deafness, cortical blindness, or symptomatic amnesias. It may also express the psychic recognition of the hostility of relatives. Anomic behavior and self-neglect can represent gradual increase in confusion and weakness from remediable or irremediable causes. Sometimes this loss of ability to tend oneself is compounded by personal pride, which makes the patient unwilling to let others see him or her in a neglected condition. The idea that old people are more commonly lonely than young, except after bereavement, may well be exaggerated as a cause of depression. Where isolation and depression coexist in the old, the isolation and neglect are more commonly results of endogenous depression than causes of reactive depression.

Paranoia in age should be distinguished from well-founded anger, frustration, and suspicion of relatives. As at any age, paranoiac ideas serve to fill gaps in the patient's ability to explain experience. They make sense of the senseless. In old age, such ideas tend to be domestic rather than extravagant, and the blanks they fill are due to sensory or cortical deficit. People are stealing the mail (since the patient writes no letters, or his friends are dead, he gets none). People are putting dirt in the washing machine (to which the patient forgot to add soap).

The first therapeutic sign is to correct sensory deficits and to detect neurological signs if any exist. Deafness notoriously predisposes. Paranoiac ideas may be part of a valiant mechanism of denial directed against apraxia, aprosopognosia, or cortical blindness, which the patient may vehemently deny (Anton's syndrome). Here, as always, one must listen carefully to what the patient says. Bizarre experiences such as temporal lobe auras, which would be recognized in younger people for what they are, may be attributed to paranoia in the old. Reports of odd behavior should be evaluated skeptically: Relatives and nurses often see as paranoid in the old behavior that in the young would be tolerated. Hidden physical determinants should be sought, such as sensory loss, tinnitus, olfactory hallucinations. The paranoid symptoms and the attendant panic may then be controlled by major tranquilizers, in low doses; since paranoid patients are paranoid about pills and may conceal them under the denture for subsequent disposal, the dose should be in liquid form. Medication must be frank, not surreptitious, or the paranoia will be reinforced with fears of poisoning or ideas of influence. In view of possible hypotensive effects, specific warning must be given for care in getting out of bed during the night and on waking. The complications of prolonged phenothiazine administration in the old include glaucoma, acute retention, extrapyramidal syndrome, and the aggravation of pre-existing tremorless parkinsonism; yet the relief of paranoia is an indication for their cautious use.

Acute and chronic anxiety reactions and panic states in the old can occur in response to any crisis, but they are specifically associated with a move to unfamiliar surroundings,[6] whether this be to hospital, to a new location, or particularly to an apartment that is a mirror image of one they have left. Most of us have experienced confusion on waking in an unfamiliar hotel room. In old age this is compounded by fear of senility and by sedation; the loss of time orientation normal to persons in hospital and separated from clocks and calendars can be read as "dementia" in the old. Such panic states respond to normal crisis intervention, sharing, suggestion of coping strategies, and reassurance coupled with help in relearning the environment. So-called minor tranquilizers may be given for 1 to 7 days only and in minimal doses.

Sleep patterns in the old are characterized by reduction in Stage 3 sleep; frequent awakening, after which sleep is resumed; and the occasional daily nap. The typical pattern of normal sleep in old age has figured widely in hypnotic advertisements under the label "geriatric insomnia." It should not be medicated, and staff who awaken older persons from daytime naps should be controlled. The physician should be aware that, with the possible exception of chloral hydrate in pediatric doses over short periods, there is no hypnotic that does not induce some degree of hangover in older subjects; and apparent dementia occasionally responds dramatically to withdrawal of a cherished sleeping pill. Barbiturates in particular can readily induce microsomal enzyme changes with consequent derangement of calcium metabolism and "senile rickets" presenting as loss of mobility and weakness. Patients and relatives need to be cautioned against over-the-counter medications that are based on hyoscine and an antihistamine; the effects of these in the old can be spectacularly deleterious and diagnostically perplexing if not recognized.

Alcohol, our chief and most threatening drug of abuse,

presents problems in old patients as at all ages. Old people "become alcoholic" because of the long latency of confrontation with an alcohol problem, because their tolerance to alcohol declines, and because they abuse alcohol for the first time in age to soften intolerable circumstances and loss of social roles. Others are given drams by relatives to keep them quiet. Alcohol has been lauded in geriatric psychiatry as a "miracle drug" for palliating the distress of age.[7] Although the reasons behind this view are clearly argued, to those obliged to deal with its effects, this kind of assertion belongs to the realm of massive social denial that surrounds the subject generally. It would perhaps be true if alcohol, like cocaine, were a controlled substance. For those brought up in the context of this denial, and of the mythology of "social" drinking, permission to continue in a style they have known is valuable.[8] On the other hand, alcoholism in old age requires active treatment as it does at any other age, and old people need to be warned of the increased susceptibility to falls and to hangover effects that even lifelong moderation cannot obviate. More than ever, the older person needs to keep his head together.

Senile dementia is the layperson's image of old age, and the fear of this destiny does much to pattern gerontophobia in society. It is significant, if not epidemic, affecting about 4.4% of persons over 65. The term covers a number of organic diseases characterized by slowly progressive loss of mental capacity, including memory, orientation, and the ability to perform serial tasks. The two leading forms in this continuum are so-called atherosclerotic dementia, which reflects not so much decreased blood flow to the brain as it does the effect of multiple successive small infarcts; and the Alzheimer group, in which cell loss is prominent. Neither is due to age alone. The infarctive syndrome may possibly be reduced in future age groups by judicious antihypertensive therapy in middle life (and can be precipitated, or aggravated, by injudicious antihypertensive therapy in old age). The Alzheimer group are probably infective or autoimmune in origin. Compared with the downward sawtooth course of infarctive dementias, that of the Alzheimer group is more smoothly progressive. Drugs have been developed that appear to palliate the course of these conditions;[9] the infarctive form sometimes responds to anticoagulant therapy with partial reversal or arrest. In either case social and environment enrichment can enable the patient to live better with the capacity he/she has. The differential diagnosis includes depressive pseudodementia; symptomatic confusion; such specific cerebral disorders as normotensive hydrocephalus; and the effects of medication. The most important pseudodementia seen among the American old is "nursing home disease," a combination of social deprivation, lack of demand, boredom, and chemical restraint by overdoses of tranquilizers given for the convenience of untrained staff and to prevent complaint. This syndrome, which resembles that seen in psychiatrically committed dissidents living in less fortunate political orders, is remediable by withdrawal of medication and restitution of social responsibilities. Untreated, it passes rapidly into the irremediable dementia that it simulates.

Active treatment of apparent dementia is always justified —whether the means be therapeutic trial of antidepressants, milieu therapy, or trial of drugs—in view of the course of the untreated disease. Removal of depressive overlay and the mobilization of social interest and intellectual reserves laid fallow by boredom can sometimes effect surprising revivals. At worst the patient can be helped to live within his cerebral means and be given a warm and supportive environment. The need for human contact persists so long as touch can be appreciated and after the loss of memory for faces.

TESTING THE MENTAL CAPACITY OF THE OLD

An old person subjected to mental testing is defensive. Aware of the social expectation of senility, less accustomed to what appears pointless exercises than the IQ-ridden generations that grew up after them, and easily time-stressed, the old approach mental tests in much the same frame of mind as a solitary black pupil in a school full of hostile whites whose teacher has prefaced the exercise with a racist discourse on the mental superiority of Anglo-Saxons. That they need to be reassured is an understatement: The magnitude of the increment in scores after administration of a beta-blocking agent[10] is concrete evidence of this need.

Slowing of the majority of physical responses is a normal consequence of age. Normal old people do not operate quickly, and they react badly to time stress, taking refuge in confusion or negativism. It is a privilege of age to close the door. Many a hearing aid has been ordered because on the day of the audiometrist's visit the patient was not talking to anyone. In modern society with its high informational flux, old people may be chronically hustled to the point of confusion, and any task used in testing must be modified time-wise to exclude the spurious case of underperformance.

Since confusion is so often symptomatic, it must be looked for in every geriatric examination. On the other hand, a healthy older person confronted on admission by a doctor young enough to be his son, who asks him whether he knows what year it is, and who is the president, can be pardoned for terminating cooperation at that point. Orientation can be determined in a wholly unthreatening manner, however, since many items of the standard Hodkinson[1] short inventory come within the scope of normal case taking: name, age, birthplace, address, name of next of kin, occupation or former occupation—even the time of the appointment, the name of the physician, and the time of day. The patient can be asked to remember an address or phrase for 5-minute recall; other essential tests, such as counting backward, are best incorporated into the physical CNS examination. Only if disorientation appears on this inventory need its extent be pursued; both mental state and the presence and nature of aphasia or memory defect can be established from conversation. When they have been cited by relatives, they can be referred to the patient in specific questions. Occasional episodes of confusion are terrifying and are likely to be volunteered, whereas even the apparently caring narration of relatives should be viewed with insightful skepticism.

In fact, the physician's examination of the old, like his response to an avowedly homosexual patient, merits close self-examination. If it is based on unrecognized hostile or patronizing attitudes, then these will be projected however bland the approach, for the nerves of the old are as raw to perceive prejudice as are those of any persecuted minority. It is helpful, perhaps, to recall the following: An old person is and feels like the same person that he/she was when young. Others are seen to age, but not we ourselves; and it is the response of others that changes from valuation to devaluation, from conventional social respect to impatience. Conversation proceeds as if the old person were not there. Waiters will ask, not the patient, but the son or daughter, "Does he take cream in his coffee?" So while we remain inwardly as we were, our surroundings and our juniors increasingly treat us as objects. The physician who not only knows but empathizes this and projects his empathy will pratice geriatric psychiatry with success. It is, after all, reasonable to work on these nosogenic attitudes in society if only to protect ourselves after we grow old.

THE DOCTOR AND "SENILITY"

"Senility" is the gradual loss of mental or physical function and well being when this occurs in an elderly person. Its distinction from general ill health depends upon the erroneous belief that age in itself is a sufficient explanation of such changes. In fact, as Hodkinson[1] points out, "senility" is to the geriatrician what "failure to thrive" is to the pediatrician; this in itself is evidence of something wrong that calls for active investigation. In view of the prevalence of genetic diseases revealing themselves in babies, and the rarity of their first appearance in old age, unexplained ill health is far more commonly "idiopathic" in pediatric than in geriatric practice. The attitude of prescientific medicine to the major infectious diseases of infancy in some respects resembled the attitude that considers senility a diagnosis, in that it attributed to "age" (in that case infancy) phenomena that in adults would be recognized as specific pathologies. In the case of the old, these are specific pathologies in which the signs and symptoms of "textbook" medicine, which is predominantly the medicine of adult and middle life, are muted or altered by aging and obscured by the persisting misconception that disability can be attributed to chronology alone.

Old people do not in fact become weak, frail, immobile, or demented through any common or near-universal change coupled to chronological age in the way that loss of hair pigment is coupled. Their liability to pathologies, and in particular multiple pathologies, increases, and although 75% of persons over 65 describe themselves as "well," about 86% suffer from one or more chronic conditions, which may be minor in their impact on function; and the 10% to 15% who are seriously "unwell" commonly have more than one such condition. In these evidently ill patients senility is no more than a slightly derogatory term for the physical and mental concomitants of chronic and explainable ill health. When it presents alone, and in the absence of any such history, it means an ongoing loss of function from an occult cause, which in a younger person would lead to intensive investigation, but in the old is treated as something to be expected. The main achievement of geriatric medicine, and the main requirement of its effective practice on the European model, is the liquidation of this erroneous belief.

How Senility Presents

Senility is not a complaint of the patient but a report by relatives or custodians of an old person. The patient may complain of weakness, loss of activity and well-being, or confusion, attributing these changes to age. In either event the factual basis is that a change in the patient has made it impossible to do what he/she recently did. In popular usage senility refers to loss of intellectual function or even to resentful or inconvenient behavior that, however justified by the setting, can be charitably attributed to such loss.

The office presentation of senility varies greatly. The following case history provides a good example:

> The father of a distinguished geriatrician was an active and feisty old man in his mid-80s, twice a widower, and a wayward pursuer of his own concerns. His son was notified by an alarmed family that Dad was "failing." He sat in a chair, he no longer showed interest in women or in food. More seriously he had three times parked his car, forgotten where he had parked it, and reported it stolen. On the first two occasions the police were tolerant; on the third they suggested that the patient might have outlived his eligibility for a driving license. A local practitioner diagnosed "old age." On examination, the old man was rational but a little confused, and the fire had gone out of him. He was also losing weight and experiencing fatigue on moving about.

I will return to this case in a moment, because the outcome is instructive. The patient was fortunate in having a geriatrician in the family; in less affluent or less supportive circumstances he would have risked admission to a custodial institution, sedation in response to his anger at the procedure, and early death from medical neglect or the civilized equivalent of black magic. That is a not uncommon outcome of symptomatic disorientation in the old when senility is treated as a diagnosis, the Shakespearean "last act."

This popular reading of senility covers the actual symptoms of confusion and memory loss, hostile or difficult behavior, and dementia, which point to wholly different probable causes. But equally common modes of presentation are weakness and loss of mobility in the absence of obvious cause such as arthritic pain (often described as "getting frail" or "going off his feet"); fatigue; and a general lack of appetency, including anorexia, loss of interest in events, and "giving up" on life (again often charitably interpreted by relatives as a fitting and even natural preparation for the cue to leave the stage). Often the onset of this downward slope in the life of the patient is presaged by a series of unexplained falls ("premonitory falls" in geriatric parlance); these may represent not only neurological disorders such as unrecognized parkinsonism or ingravescent stroke, but also constitute a common presentation in advanced age of heart attack, heart failure, chest or urinary infection, or the equally ingravescent side effects of medication.

The common thread in all these "senile" manifestations is that in old age the presentation of major illness is commonly nonspecific. Moreover the popular reading of senility as "second-childishness" cannot be separated from the physical pathologies that occur in age, because confusion, memory loss, and behavioral and mood changes are increasingly often symptomatic in older patients, as delirium is symptomatic of febrile illness in the young—the difference being that at advanced ages they may be the only symptoms.

"Senility" as a Mental Symptom

The commonest psychiatric disorders of old age are not "senile dementias" (meaning organic and structural loss of brain function) but symptomatic clouding of consciousness and endogenous depression with approximately equal frequency. Endogenous depression in the old may present as hypochondria or pseudodementia, may be accompanied by a loss of activity and mental grasp, and may itself rapidly impair physical health. It is also treatable by appropriate antidepressant therapy. Symptomatic confusion, memory loss, or agitation can result from any silent infection, cerebrovascular or coronary occlusion, electrolyte disturbance from any cause, and the effects of medication. In contrast to the major organic dementias, these symptomatic changes are often (though not always) less gradual in onset, and they are transient if the cause is removed before grave physical and social damage has been done. The major disease process may differ from its typical adult form in being painless (coronary occlusion), afebrile (pneumonia, pyelitis), and attended by minimal signs.

Symptomatic mental illness in the old, whether it presents as memory loss, acute confusion, or apathy, is usually recognized for what it is when it occurs in the presence of obvious illness. Unfortunately this is often not the case. Mental symptoms of what is in fact minor delirium presenting as the only evidence of disorder can be the first or sole evidence of pneumonia, urinary infection, uremia, congestive heart failure, minor cerebral infarction without other gross neurological signs, diabetic ketosis or hypoglycemia, and hypothermia (older persons living in cold areas and inadequate housing are especially prone to the latter). In all these cases, the myth of senility may lead the incautious to miss the underlying pathology; this is a serious matter, because where the pathology is treatable, mental function usually returns completely. So long as the mental association between age and dementia persists, the minimal increase in respiratory rate of afebrile pneumonia or the presence of urinary infection can be missed. The diagnosis of Valium (diazepam) deficiency and other injudicious interventions directed to quieten the "demented" patient can add to the mischief. Institutionalization in a custodial "home" is in itself a potent cause of nocturnal confusion, especially in the already sick, and the treatment of this by chemical restraint constitutes an unintentional form of euthanasia in a patient whose mental confusion might have been curable had the diagnostician had minimal geriatric training.

Next to infection, the commonest cause of senility presenting with confusion is medication. For this reason the first step to take in its investigation is the "plastic bag test" mentioned above. The second step is the cessation of all such medication that is not life-sustaining. Let me go back to the case history I cited above.

The geriatrician's father received a careful physical examination, which revealed no sign of infection or any other of the common physical causes of his condition. He denied taking any medication. Diligent inquiry, however, revealed that at the death of his first wife many years before, he had been unable to sleep, and since that time he had taken a single butabarbital tablet every night. When his second wife had died, 5 years previously, he again could not sleep, and added a single nightly Quaalude (methaqualone) tablet. This trifling amount of medication was stopped, over his protests. Within 10 days his activity and appetency returned, he ate well, pursued comely women, and never again mislaid his car. His strength and posture also greatly improved with the removal of mild osteomalacia due to the microsomal-inductive effect of the barbiturate, from which he had been suffering.

Senile Weakness

Physical strength, in athletic terms, normally declines with age, but such a decline is also normally gradual. The patient adjusts to it; thus, weakness of rapid onset, similar to that which is experienced in earlier life after a severe illness, is always symptomatic. It may cover increasing dyspnea or clinically predictable conditions such as anemia, but in the old other less familiar causes may operate. The weakness of spontaneous or drug-induced osteomalacia ("senile rickets") is one such cause. Another is the myopathy of silent hyperthyroidism ("apathetic" thyrotoxicosis). Sodium depletion—either renal or, more commonly, iatrogenic, from the use of diuretics, heart failure, and silent coronary infarction—can also present as weakness. It can also represent polymyalgia rheumatica, the stiffness of tremorless parkinsonism, and other pathologies, including malignancy.

Treatment of hypertension in old people, if the physician misguidedly attempts to lower the blood pressure to a "young" norm, can precipitate senility via electrolyte loss, and it can also cause hypotensive falls, impotency, and a whole range of iatrogenic mischief, including decreased cerebral function.

Senile Memory Loss

Like many other responses, recall gets slower with age. This effect, which troubled Thomas Jefferson and led him to argue against a life presidency, is most prominent in those least mentally active, but causes most anxiety to the intellectual. It is benign and nonprogressive, however. Severe deterioration of memory can herald the major dementias, but equally common or commoner causes are undiagnosed myxedema and hangover due to the use, even in normally acceptable doses, of any sedative drug. There are no "minor tranquilizers" in geriatrics; nor should the normal later-life pattern of light sleep and frequent waking be medicated, although it needs to be distinguished from the early waking characteristic of depressive illness.

The Investigation of "Senility"

The investigation of senility resolves itself into the careful search for the underlying pathology; the removal of iatrogenic disease where present; and the healing, in patient, relatives, and the physician himself, of the sorcery wrought by the assumption of causeless infirmity as a feature of old age.

The minimal exclusionary approach to senility involves a proper history; a full physical exmination carried out with patience (no simple matter where confusion or deafness limit cooperation) with special attention to infections and to the signs, often minimal, of endocrine and metabolic disorder; and a battery of tests directed to the known causes of nonspecific illness. For such a battery Hodkinson[1] suggests chest x-ray, with attention to signs of infection, pulmonary edema, neoplasm, and bony changes, including fractures and Looser's zones in the scapula; Coulter S blood count; BUN and electrolytes; serum albumin and globulin; calcium, phosphates, and alkaline phosphatase; a random blood sugar; T4 and T3 uptake; and routine urinalysis. To these should be added thorough inquiry into, and re-evaluation of, all medications without exception. This latter should be carried out with reference to a geriatric textbook, not the maker's literature, since the list of precautions and side effects required by the FDA contains no special reference to drug hazards in age. All medication not evidently life-sustaining may well be withdrawn, with due attention to possible effects of sudden discontinuance and interaction of retained with withdrawn drugs, e.g., through loss of ribosomal induction. When investigation is complete and symptoms have remitted or been explained, only those medications should be reinstated which are clearly indicated, and those should not exceed four or five in number, however numerous the pathologies identified. Sedatives, antihypertensives, and diuretics are the most abused drugs in older persons. They are rarely or never indicated for prolonged use.

GERIATRIC TRAINING

It is sometimes argued that geriatrics is not a subject, and that the care of the old is within the competence of any good internist. In theory this is perhaps true, in that the care of the old falls best within the scope of the primary care physician. Geriatric specialists are of value in hospitals and in the creation of teaching centers, but the further fragmentation of general medicine is not desirable. On the other hand, deans of medical schools who reject the teaching of geriatrics as a special accessory skill are reflecting their own lack of awareness of shortcomings: It would be interesting to subject both them and their students to an elementary quiz in geriatric medicine.

The lack of specific training in geriatrics at all in but a very few American schools raises the possibility of an unwelcome scenario; First, new health care legislation exposes the lack of geriatricians; then physicians lacking in geriatric experience attempt to meet this need; and finally, unsatisfactory results lead to the despoiling of European geriatric services for trained staff. There is indeed nothing in the factual base of geriatrics that cannot be acquired from the excellent European textbooks, such as those of Hodkinson[1] or Brocklehurst,[10] but the bases of both geriatric knowledge and physician interest are attitudinal; and to inspire these, as well as the exchange of European experience, a program of exchange fellowships is urgently needed. In particular the growing interest in geriatric psychiatry will depend for success on expert geriatric medicine, since its patients exhibit both the physical effects of "ageism" in society and the symptomatic syndromes that increasingly affect mental state in later life. In testing these physician skills, the approach to reported "senility" is critical, and this test is one that both the student now in training and the practitioner aiming at higher effectiveness should consciously prepare to meet.

REFERENCES

1. Hodkinson, H. M. *Common symptoms of disease in the elderly.* Oxford: Blackwell, 1976.

2. Finch, C. E. The regulation of physical changes during mammalian aging. *Quarterly Review of Biology, 51,* 49–83, 1976.

3. Linn, L. Clinical manifestations of psychiatric disorders. In *Comprehensive Textbook of Psychiatry,* Vol. 1. Freedman, A. M., Kaplan, H. I., & Sadock, B. J. (Eds.). Baltimore: William & Wilkins, 1975.

4. Hall, P. Differential diagnosis and treatment of depression in the elderly. *Gerontologia Clinica, 16,* 1–3; 126–136, 1974.

5. Foster, J. R., Gershell, W. J., & Goldfarb, A. I. Lithium treatment for the elderly. I. Clinical usage. *Journal of Gerontology, 32,* 299–302, 1977.

6. Hall, P., Clinical aspects of moving house as a precipitant of psychiatric symptoms. *Journal of Psychosomatic Research, 10,* 59–80, 1966.

7. Stotsky, B. A. Psychoactive drugs for geriatric patients with psychiatric disorders. In *Aging 2: Genesis and treatment of psychologic disorders in the elderly.* Gershon, S., & Raskin, A. (Eds.). New York: Raven Press, 1975, pp. 252–253.

8. Chien, C. P., Stotsky, B. A., & Cole, J. O. Psychiatric treatment for nursing-home patients: drug, alcohol and milieu. *American Journal of Psychiatry, 130,* 543–548, 1973.

9. Lehmann, H. E., & Ban, T. CNS stimulants and anabolic substances. In *Aging: Genesis and treatment of psychologic disorders in the elderly.* Gershon, S., & Raskin, A. (Eds.). New York: Raven Press, 1975, pp. 179–202.

10. Brocklehurst, J. C. *Textbook of geriatric medicine and gerontology.* London: Churchill, Second Edition, 1979.

Chapter 4

GERONTOLOGICAL NURSING
Virginia Stone

I should like, first of all, to make clear the distinction between medical care and nursing care. To illustrate the distinction, the activities of the physician, the nurse, and the social worker are described as three separate circles.

Each of these professions has independent functions as well as interindependent functions. This means that there is an overlapping of these circles of performance, and it becomes difficult to say that one particular activity is nursing; another is medicine; or still another is social work. On occasion, one can identify areas specific to nursing, but at other times there is an overlapping with one or both other professions. Such overlap is probably true of most disciplines, even in areas such as sociology, psychology, and social psychology. There is, for example, the question as to where social psychology should fall: under sociology, psychology, or independently. This is equally true of the health and medical professions.

Although definitions of medicine, nursing, or social work can be troublesome, a somewhat succinct and simple definition can be arrived at. Nursing is any act performed by a nurse, and medicine is any act performed by a physician. The same is true of social work.

There is an outstanding task force report called *The Future of Long Term Care in the United States,* which was released in February of 1977. The task force was composed of social workers who described as one of the dilemmas of delivering services to the elderly, the lack of viable, cohesive relationships among mutually related systems. The task force regarded this as a major impediment to the development of a continuum of care for persons at risk.

The caring professions should have sufficiently matured by now, so that we should not be fighting over turf. Rather, we should be giving what we have the knowledge to give in order to perform the best service necessary for the aging.

In order to provide some framework for the discussion to follow, it is necessary to consider nursing in relation to the process of aging and the needs of the older person. Nursing should strive to provide those needs at the level of promotion, prevention, maintenance, and restoration of health. If this is done, then we cannot speak of ourselves as geriatric nurses, but we must speak of ourselves as gerontological nurses.

Geriatrics deals with illness, as does geriatric nursing. Gerontological nursing deals with the process of aging; those who have been following some of the trends lately know that there are many who now feel that functional state of the individual—of the aged—takes precedence over medical diagnosis. This means that in order to meet the needs of the older person, we must first know the functional state; the disease part can come second. To say someone has cancer, for example, tells you little about the individual. One individual with cancer may be well and functioning fully, while another may be terminally ill. Another disease entity that is common among older people is diabetes. The diagnosis alone tells little about the person; we must know more about the functional ability.

Functional state refers to both physical and mental states.

Unfortunately, for many persons the functional state means solely the physical state.

When reference is made to the gerontological nurse, such perception must be based upon a broader frame of reference than that of geriatric nursing practice. Many factors have direct bearing upon recent developments in gerontological nursing, but three principal factors deserve particular attention. The gerontological nurse is influenced by professional shifts in the changing roles of the professional nurse. A second shift influencing her/him is that of population change or population shift. And the third one is that of political shifts. Much of what the gerontological nurse will be able to do will depend on the power in the political arena.

THE INCREASING OLDER POPULATION AND THE GERONTOLOGICAL NURSE

Let us examine the influence of the population shifts on gerontological nursing, bearing in mind that persons 75 and older are among the fastest growing segment of the United States population. In the year 2000, half of the 65-and-over group will be 75 and over, with 11% being 85 and over. Approximately 42% of those who are 75 and over have substantial limitations in such activities as walking, climbing, and bending.

Because of this tremendous increase in persons aged 75 and over, a great deal of study is being done in the United States concerning the frail elderly, as this has become an area of great concern. Three major documents were recently issued dealing with the frail elderly. One of the reports, issued by the National Academy of Science and titled *A policy statement: the elderly and functional dependence,* states that "functional dependent elderly are defined as those individuals over 65 whose illnesses, impairments, and social problems have become disabling, reducing their ability to carry out independently the customary activities of daily life." Functional dependency is more prevalent in those age 75 and over, and, therefore, the statement addresses itself to this age group.

The committee that made this report was guided in its deliberations by two basic principles:

1. The care of the elderly should be directed toward the maintenance of maximum possible functional social independence.
2. Health care and social services should be provided in a manner that preserves the dignity of the elderly individual and provides opportunity for personal choice.

It is recognized that the care of the functionally dependent elderly person requires a different orientation toward patient outcomes than prevails in the care of acute illness or trauma. It is believed that the future needs for care of the older person can be found through more intensive assessment of those aged 75 and over.

Another statement indicating concern for the frail elderly was the recommendation from the Federal Council of Aging to the president of the United States. This report reiterates some of the same concerns evidenced in the statement cited earlier. The caretaker role, however, is more explicitly identified in the report of the Federal Council on Aging. The needs of this group are further identified in the budget issue paper, *Long term care for the elderly and disabled.*

All three of these reports have been routed to the office of the president. What will now happen to these reports in relation to their reaching the Congress is questionable and dependent upon the president.

NEED FOR HEALTH ASSESSMENT

A common thread found in all three recommendations lies in the need for health assessment, with recognition that such should be available for all older people at the government's expense, on a voluntary basis. These reports also indicate that such assessment should begin with the frail elderly, those aged 75 and over. Although the need for health assessment is great among all older people, the frail elderly have so many needs that we should begin with this group and then move down the age scale. With health assessment in focus, then, we must ask what it is, what it does, and where should it be done.

The health assessment referred to in the reports mentioned earlier is far more inclusive than a general medical examination or medical history. Several items important in health assessment of the older person that may not be a routine part of a medical history or examination require explication in greater detail.

One of the first things we have to do in health assessment of the aged is determine where the individual is on the continuum of aging in relation to the sensory processes. We cannot satisfactorily communicate with the individual until we have tested his/her ability to hear or to discriminate speech. Although our methods for assessing the sensory processes are gross, they do give us some kind of understanding of where the individual is on the continuum of aging. It is interesting to note that in Texas a manual is now being developed for testing the sensory processes. This is a growing concern. It is difficult to understand, however, why it is that we have special people going out to perform such tests, when such tests can easily be incorporated as a part of health assessment by nurses.

Another part of health assessment that is not often included in the history is that of the life-style of the individual. In providing care we have a responsibility to preserve the life-style of the individual, unless there is some reason for modification for the good of that individual. Often we modify a life-style to suit the convenience of the institution or the worker; but we cannot be certain as to what kind of modification is needed unless we have a more complete history of the individual's life-style. As a specific example, we can refer to postural hypotension. Some postural hypotension is related to movement out of bed. If we know that the individual is confused upon arising in the morning, we might suspect that he had a sudden drop in blood pressure because of his pattern of getting out of bed. Therefore, we would have the responsibility of teaching him about slow movement in relation to his blood pressure drop, which would be a modification in his life pattern.

A third fact in health assessment should be an awareness of the individual's understanding of his health problem, and his expectations in relation to this. As illustration, one old gentleman was very much upset because his expectations were that he would die. He expected to die because he had a urinary catheter. His interpretation of a urinary catheter was that he would have to have surgery. Since he was too old to have surgery, he was certain that he would die. When someone realized his lack of understanding of a urinary catheter and provided him with proper information, his expectations were changed.

Importance of Baseline Data

One of the things that is so very important in health assessment is the collection of baseline data to determine the individual's average. Reference here is to data that we collect every day but fail to utilize to its fullest potential, such as temperature, pulse, respiration, and blood pressure. In health assessment we often do not identify the baseline data and their meaning to the health behavior of older people.

These are major conditions in caring for older people. We cannot stress enough the importance of knowing the average blood pressure range in the standing, sitting, and the lying position of the individual. Until we have those data, we are not ready to evaluate falls in blood pressure. A fall in blood pressure from prolonged sitting is an interesting example: How do we know that the blood pressure has dropped due to the pooling of blood in the abdomen unless we have baseline data from which to make such a judgment?

Another of the areas in which we have limited knowledge,

is in determining what is the normal range of temperature for older people. This is one of the areas where we need tremendous amounts of research. We know, in general, that many older people have a normal temperature that is lower than what is usually considered to be normal temperature. Thus we need to know the average range of temperature for a particular individual, in order to properly interpret a rise in temperature.

Social Components

These are just very simple things that we need to take into consideration in health assessment if we are going to provide quality intervention. Health assessment must also include social components. Social workers in their report, to which I alluded earlier, are recommending that there be a social health model. In fact, they looked at the SHMO as a model for assessment of older people, in that it incorporates both social and health aspects. In the work conducted by Eric Pfeiffer in his OARS scale, he has included quite a bit of material with respect to social, as well as mental and physical health.

Also, in such health assessment we need to gather more information about support systems. What kind of support systems have worked? What kinds are available? And what kinds do we need? This is particularly crucial in decisions relating to the individual's ability to remain in the community, rather than his being institutionalized. If we did much more assessment of the support system, then it might be possible to keep more older people in the community.

OPTIMAL CONDITIONS FOR HEALTH ASSESSMENT

There is always the big question in all of these reports as to who should do the patient assessment. Social workers might be saying, "Oh, I can do that"; and nurses certainly feel, "I can do it"; and very likely some doctors feel, "This is my job." As a result, we do not get, through the reports, any guidance as to which particular groups should be engaged in health assessment. Several of them are recommending that health assessment be on a team basis composed of a physician, a nurse, and a social worker. There are some demonstrations going, especially in the mountain states, using the team approach in health assessment.

It appears, and this may well be professional bias, that the gerontological nurse could be the health assessor. A good health assessor would know when to refer the individual for further assessment to one of the other disciplines. Whoever does the health assessment, however, must do it in a systematic way. We have diligently been trying to develop scales that would provide assessment in a systematic way. Each of the scales that have been tried has strengths and weaknesses. No single such scale has been approved as the one to be used throughout the country. Perhaps none ever will be.

It is also important to consider where health assessment might be done. From the gerontological nursing point of view, it would seem that gerontological nursing should be delivered wherever older people are located, such as in the senior centers, the day care centers, private homes, and nursing homes. Unfortunately, this is not where the gerontological nurse is to be found.

We find a limited number of nurses in senior centers or day care centers or delivering home care. We find more in the nursing home, but this is still a small number of nurses in relation to the number of patients in nursing homes. For example, we have at the present time more nursing home beds in the United States than we have general hospital beds. Where are all the nurses? The reply is obvious. But the gerontological nurse is not where the majority of older people are.

There is a movement toward designating the senior centers as the focal point of delivery of health care to the elderly, since the senior center activity in this country will be developed to a greater extent than it is now. Before Arthur Flemming retired as commissioner of the Administration on Aging, he was advocating this. The new commissioner has had a great deal of experience in the senior centers, and there is reason to believe that he will continue this interest. The nurse has a tremendous role to play in the senior centers. At the outset, senior centers adopted the social model, and the health model was largely absent. If we can bring together the two models, the SHMO, we can offer more comprehensive service to the older person.

It is amazing and gratifying to observe the variety of tasks undertaken by students placed in senior centers. They are proving to be tremendous counselors. One of the areas in which they are functioning is that of coordinator of patient care, because many of the people attending senior centers are going to multiple physicians. For example, one individual was going to two physicians, each of whom had prescribed diuretics. Consequently, she was getting a double dosage of diuretics for the lack of a coordinator of her care. It would appear that the nurse has a tremendous role to play in the senior center as coordinator.

We have a new senior center opening in our area, and a new high-rise apartment building. Over 300 elderly people will be moving into the high-rise. Each of these people will receive health assessment by gerontological nurses. From these health assessments, we hope to be able to determine what the health program should be for the high-rise apartment complex. Through such an approach, we can develop a program that will meet the needs of these specific people in that space.

The day care centers are also rapidly springing up around this country. These also offer tremendous opportunity for gerontological nursing care. Not only can the nurse give individual care, but she can serve as a consultant to the total staff.

We need to remember that in both the day care centers and senior centers, we have large numbers of indigenous workers who are there because of different federal programs. The senior aide often is a good person, but is just as often an untrained person. There are instances where the personnel is simply not qualified to carry on the responsibilities that the job calls for.

As a result, within day care and senior centers we often have a large group of well-meaning persons who have very limited backgrounds on the aged. The nurse who has a background in gerontological nursing can thus act in a consultant capacity for a number of these workers. Also, the nurse in the day care center has a tremendous opportunity to work with families to enable them to understand the 24-hour needs of the individuals.

Working with the families of people who utilize the day care centers has been one of the most gratifying experiences for nursing students. Students have been engaged in teaching health care to groups of participants. Some of the health care interests expressed by those groups included discussions of nerves, headaches, and operations. One topic that surfaced during a discussion was cataract surgery. One of the people had had cataract surgery, while another was about to have it. The exchange and support between these persons was outstanding.

When given the opportunity to express their needs, older people in day care centers, senior centers, and the like, will suggest areas in which they need more knowledge that might have totally escaped the attention of health care providers, if such selections were left totally to them.

The role of the nurse in the home care program is of great interest to gerontological nurses. The whole home care movement has suffered great neglect in the United States. Historically, some of the first home care programs were developed at the turn of the century; but home care has never really flourished in the United States. The only time that it flourished at all was when the Metropolitan Life Insurance Company was paying for home care, and they were able to sell their policies on the basis of home care, especially with the delivery of babies at home. Another time was during the Red Cross Town and Country Program. All in all, however rare, there have been some examples of outstanding home care programs in the United States, principally in the large cities. Although home care has been with us for over 75 years, it has not flourished; nor has home care kept pace with the needs of older people.

As Ethel Shanas has sufficiently documented, there are more sick people at home than there are in institutions. If this is indeed the case, it is difficult to comprehend why we concentrate our nursing care in the institution rather than in homes. Part of this is due, of course, to the lack of reimbursement or insufficient reimbursement. Nonetheless, the nurse has a major role in developing home care. Perhaps as she moves into her new professional role as gerontological nurse, she will be more independent in determining who needs home care.

In the area of nursing homes, we do have nurses moving into that sphere, but not in sufficient numbers. The role of the gerontological nurse may well differ from that traditionally assigned her. The regulation requiring a medical director in nursing homes raises interesting professional questions. Concern has been expressed with respect to the quality of the medical directors, across the board, in nursing homes. It may well be that we should look at a different model, that the gerontological nurse should be the manager of patient care, and the physician should assume a consultant role.

This is not a new pattern, for the Loeb Center in New York has experimented with this very successfully over a number of years. We have, however, been slow in adopting this method. If we are really going to improve the care of the patient, we must have a different model, and the model we may need to consider is that of the nurse as the manager of patient care.

IMPORTANCE OF TEACHING SELF-ASSESSMENT

Another area that we need to look at, a growing area of concern, is in teaching older people self-assessment. There is a growing interest in the country in teaching various age groups self-assessment. The older person needs this as much as, if not more than, any other age group. For we know that in certain cultures some older people delay seeking medical help until there is acute pain: That is their orientation. If older persons could be taught more self-assessment and the danger signs, then they would more likely have a better opportunity for early diagnosis, and they would change their pattern of seeking medical care. It would be interesting to see, for example, how great an increase there would be in the number of pap smears done on older people, if older people could do them themselves, rather than having to go to somebody else for this test. There is no guarantee that the health picture would materially change, but these are some of the things that we should look at in the near future.

Just as we are teaching younger women to do their own pelvic examinations and pap smears, we should encourage older people in such activities as well. We could teach them a great deal about blood pressure, for example, and have them assume responsibility in relation to their own blood pressure.

We already know that the individual assumes responsibility for his own health. This is a part of our way of living. What we really need to do is to provide individuals with sufficient knowledge to assume this responsibility intelligently. In order to carry this through, two great areas of need must be addressed: continuity of care and coordination. When we examine the lack of continuity and what is happening to people because of it, we cannot help but realize that we must have better methods of continuity, which means more effective coordination. Although particular reference has been made to the nurse as the coordinator of health care in the senior center, she could become the coordinator of patient care in many other kinds of settings as well.

UPGRADING THE ROLE OF THE GERONTOLOGICAL NURSE

In order to do this, one of our major concerns is to be sure that we have nurses who are well qualified for this level of performance. We are improving gerontological education in the nursing profession through the number of master's courses we provide with gerontological content. There has been educational content in dealing with the care of the aged in the undergraduate curriculum. A primary concern, however, is the qualification of the faculty to teach such material. The same concern is equally relevant to instruction in geriatrics. There is great concern on the part of many professional persons with respect to the quality of faculty teaching geriatric medicine and gerontological nursing.

Another concern is, will these people, once prepared, find employment? Because of some of the legislation and financial structure, some gerontological nurses who have gone through good programs are unable to find employment in that particular specialty. The recent Rural Health Clinic Bill affords some hope that nurses will be able to practice at a higher level and get adequate reimbursement. It is hoped that the passage of this bill will open other arenas in nursing.

Until that time we need increased research and demonstration to prove what is workable, for we are still working too much on hunches and not on the basis of sound demonstrations and research.

One of the things that continues to be rather interesting and puzzling is that after all of our experience, we have no research that tells us what should be the nurse staffing patterns in nursing homes. There are some state regulations with minimal guides. To date, we do not know what kind of mix of staff is necessary for quality care: how many LPNs, how many gerontological nurse practitioners, how many nurses' aides are needed. We have had some studies in the use of the all-professional nursing staff, however.

The Loeb Center provides one example where only the professional nurse is used. Statistics show short stays, low costs, and so forth. Another recent report, from the VA in San Antonio, Texas, describes using an all-nurse staff for patient care; this report shows that under some circumstances you can operate with an all-professional nurse staff at lower costs than using mixed staff. What we really need is to have some demonstrations and some research in this area before we can determine which pattern is best.

The area is wide open for study. One of the areas in which we really need research is in studying a group of people who comply to their drug orders, compared to a group of those who do not. We need additional data on particular populations, such as the person who is on an antihypertensive drug and takes it in relation to his/her feelings, compared to the one who complies to the requirements. Many older people do not take their antihypertensive drug regularly and instead regulate dosages in relation to their own feelings.

Another area in which research is badly needed is that of temperature range. We do not know, for example, what is the average temperature range for the older person. Some of this is very basic and very simple, but until we have good research findings on which to base our health care of older people, we will be going much by imitation and intuition. Imitation and intuition may provide good care in some instances, but it is not good enough. We must also be supported with good research.

Although the nurse has a tremendous role to play, such a role must be based on solid educational plans. The nurse must be provided with the opportunity to use her skills to the greatest extent. Functioning in this way, she may or may not be an independent practitioner. There will be many ways in which she can perform her role.

With better qualified nurses as our goal, we will be able to do a great deal towards enhancing the quality of care to ensure the older person's quality of life until death.

Part II

PSYCHOSOCIAL PROBLEMS IN LATER LIFE

Problems encountered by persons in old age are seldom either inherent in the process of aging or necessarily related to individual life-styles.

Problems that are psychosocial in nature are closely tied to attitudes, treatment procedures, societal provisions for health care, acceptance of particular caring needs of dying persons and their families, and opportunities for life enhancement. Whether such possibilities are made available to older persons largely determines their ability to function effectively and maximally within a society.

Often contrasts between nations provide the opportunity for more broadly conceiving care and services for older persons, although no system of care developed in one nation can be duplicated, without fundamental revisions, in another. The dissemination and sharing of ideas on an international scale is rapidly coming to be an effective way for nations to plan realistically for the complex network of services required to serve the elderly population adequately.

Not only is the United States an aging nation, but we participate in an aging world with other nations throughout the world. Perhaps in trying to deal with the problems faced by older persons, nations will also begin to unite through common concerns and to relate in more humanistic ways. The aging of the world may prove to be more of a unifying force than we yet recognize.

Chapter 5

DEATH AND DYING: SUPPORT SYSTEMS

Sue Cox

Hospice is a program of palliative and supportive care for terminal patients and their families. Such a program was developed in the Greater New Haven, Connecticut area in 1974, patterned after similar organizations in England, especially St. Christopher's and St. Joseph's in London, and St. Luke's in Sheffield.

One of the goals of Hospice is to help the patient to live as fully as possible; and to keep the patient in his own home, with his loved ones, for as long as this is appropriate. The emphasis is on care of the person, not just his disease. While attacking physical pain and other distressing symptoms with all of the resources of modern medicine, efforts are made to ease the mental, spiritual, and social suffering of the patient and his/her family.

The unit of care is the patient and the family. Including the family under the umbrella of care is an essential component of a program of care for dying patients. Support of the family is continued through the bereavement process.

The Hospice Home Care Team, an interdisciplinary team, consists of a paid staff of physicians, nurses, a social worker, a chaplain, a director of volunteers, a consultant physical therapist, a consultant psychiatrist, secretaries, and administrative staff. The Home Care unpaid staff (the volunteers) are nurses, homemakers, business persons, clergy, engineers, a clinical psychologist, a physician, a hairdresser, a creative movement therapist, and a person who likes to go fishing. Hospice has additional departments for public information and education, and for the planning and development of the total program.

Members of the Home Care Team make regular visits and are on call 24 hours per day, 7 days a week, to make house calls to patients on the program.

Hospice has working relationships, governed by contractual agreements, with the Visiting Nurse Association in its service area, and it works cooperatively with other components of the Greater New Haven health care delivery system.

As of May 1, 1978, 724 patients and families have received care through the full scope of services provided by the Team, plus an additional 62 patients and their families through physician or relative consultation. Fifty-seven percent of the patients have died at home.

The Hospice Home Care service area is currently eighteen towns in the Greater New Haven area; this will expand to twenty towns at the end of this year. The inpatient facility will be dedicated in October 1979. It will contain backup beds for the Home Care Program, provide inpatient beds for patients throughout Connecticut, and include a day care center for children and an outpatient clinic and offices for the Home Care Program.

Hospice is a specialized health care program emphasizing the management of pain and other symptoms associated with terminal illness. The primary goal is to control the symptoms of patients with a limited life expectancy for whom cure is no longer a reality. The goal is to enable patients to carry on an alert and pain-free existence through the careful administration of appropriate drugs and other forms of therapy, so that the patient may live fully until death.

The Hospice interdisciplinary team is but one of the units of support for dying patients and their families in the New Haven area. The other units include: the patient's physician, the public health nurse, the acute care hospital, the pharmacy, other service agencies, the family's clergyman, the circle of friends, the patient's family, and the patient. All of these units attempt to operate in a cooperative and complementary system of support for the dying patient and his family.

The patient and the family are included as a unit of the support system. The team does not think of "doing for" the patient and family but rather of "doing with" them. One of the family members was asked, at the time of discharge, how Hospice had helped. The answer was, "It's difficult to describe. We thought of you people as keeping our backbones supported, so our hands were free to do the work."

The patient and family system does need support. Americans created a problem with dying in America when we became specialized experts in disease control and cure. In many other parts of the world, people still experience dying at home, with the extended family and often the entire community participating in active roles or at least as observers. By sending disease into grand institutions full of experts and equipment—as well as rules such as short visiting hours, no children, and little family space—we have also isolated dying. Therefore, the average citizen has no experience and no role models in his/her background with which to identify.

Though much has been written, spoken, and filmed on the subject of death and dying recently, when dying comes to the typical American family, they are faced with the additional problems of being unprepared, unhelped, and often isolated; not just the patient, but loved ones, too.

My parents' end of life was not very unusual. When my father was dying in Illinois, my mother began to realize that her son lived in California, her daughter lived in Connecticut, and her friends were pulling away because they did not know what to do or what to say. She discovered that she knew nothing of their financial, insurance, or legal affairs, which her husband had handled for 50 years. She was not a nurse, so she would not know how to care for him; he was hospitalized. She did not feel it was appropriate to bother the busy nurses or doctors with questions about his illness, though she did want to know.

My mother stayed at my father's bedside every minute of visiting hours, except when the nurses had to do something to her husband, and she was asked to leave the room. She was phoned at home one night at 2:00 a.m. and told that her husband had died. After the 1 week of rituals and roles planned for participants in mourning in America, she grieved alone for 1 year, and then she died.

Across the country, the helping professions are realizing that they must be prepared to support people as they die and to help loved ones through the loss and the normal grieving process. Most institutions of higher learning are now offering courses on death and dying. Most helping professional disciplines are offering the subject at conferences and seminars. We understand the need for support.

Hospice teams are considered to be experts in the field of death and dying. We have the practical experience. We have read the current literature and taken the current courses. We understand the universal patterns and stages people must work through.

But our patients and families have taught us a most important lesson. We must not allow experience and expertise to specialize us out of the ability to care for the individual. The book has not been written yet about my dying. I am unique. I will be the expert on my dying: it has never been done before. No one is able to climb into my skin and experience my history of ethnic heritage, religious beliefs, conditioning, body chemistry. No other person can know my level of physical pain, my anxiety, my depression, unless I communicate. There are no other experts on my feelings, my hurts, my hopes.

I will be the expert on my dying. If you want to use the skills of your discipline to support me through my dying, you need, above all else, expertise in active listening. Listening for caregivers includes the skill to help people identify problems and then to communicate those areas where help is needed.

The information we need in order to support dying patients will include facts and feelings. Words frequently express neither. An effective listener will listen to the words, but also to the eyes, the body language, the family interaction, and the silence. Those of us who work in home care have the additional advantage of listening to the environment of the home.

The listener must show full attention, full acceptance, and full approval of the person's right to feel, and express facts and feelings that are true for the patient. When there is no physiological reason for a patient to be having pain, but the patient still feels pain, a physician must be prepared to help that person identify emotional, spiritual, or social suffering that can cause or exacerbate physical pain. When a lifelong religious person does not want to pray, a clergyman must listen for anger, guilt, physical pain, or the acute need for a bedpan.

The dying often get caught in systems that have personnel trained to care for the acutely ill. Consider the depth of active listening required in these two cases: To help a 30-year-old patient who is in a hospital recuperating from an appendectomy, all disciplines need a certain amount of information. To help a 30-year-old patient with terminal cancer and a prognosis of 2 months who is in the same hospital, the listening needs to cover broad areas of physical, psychological, and social concerns. Both patients might have severe pain or bouts of vomiting, and there is the hope that it will eventually lessen without drugs. Both might have a hospital bill, but only one is likely to be able to work while paying it. Both might have spouses and small children; both might have spiritual questions; both might have living parents; both might have mortgaged houses that need painting; both might have hopes to travel to Europe next year. All of these areas of concern are of a very different importance for the dying person.

It is important that we listen to the person who is acutely ill in order to treat the disease. It is essential that we listen to the person who is dying. When caring for terminal patients, it is essential that we control the symptoms of disease, and that we also listen from the perspective of treating the person.

The second message from our experience is that we will not be able to support the dying person while we are hiding from our own death. We are unable to be truly present to the suffering, anxieties, and deepest desires of the dying if these trigger uneasy feelings or open wounds we have repressed. Working with dying patients teaches us to confront our fears of our own dying and death.

The following exercise, composed of four questions, is used in training groups at Hospice. This exercise has a dual purpose: (1) to help persons to look at death; and (2) to provide the Hospice Team with a list of the corporate problems and concerns of the entire patient/family caseload.

1. If you could choose when you would die, when would it be? When would you not want to die? Why?
2. If you could choose how you would die, how would it be? How not? Why?
3. Thinking of that person with whom you are most close, who would you want to die first? Why?
4. What do you fear most about dying?

As we look at the usual answers from groups training at Hospice, we must remember that we are only trying to project; we are fantasizing. For patients and families, death has become a reality. The plans and dreams for the future are not going to be; the end of life is not coming at the chosen time, or in the chosen way! To complicate the problem list, many people have never even considered the end of life as a possibility; therefore they have the additional burden of being unprepared.

By thinking through our own feelings, we will be better equipped for trying to understand the problems and concerns of others. As a bonus, we might gain some insight into some personal priorities for the living.

For the question of when we would choose to die, most of us would not choose today, or next month, or perhaps even this year. Most of us would choose to be very old, and very old is different for different ages. Age does not seem to make a big difference. The best time to die seems to be at the end of a phase of life, and before the next goals and dreams have been realized: after I complete my education; after I get married; after my children are grown and established; after I make a significant contribution to my field; after I write my book or symphony or learn to paint; after my grandchildren are born; after they are grown; after I see my first great grandchild; after I've worked out the meaning of life; after I've fulfilled my purpose; after I know God.

Why would we not choose to die today? Most of us have a few people we need to see, a few "I love you's" to say, a few "I'm sorry's" that we have neglected. We need to get our business, financial, and legal affairs in order so as to provide for our dependents. We have always wanted to travel, to see our country and the world. Many marriages have been lived through with the anticipation of getting to know each other in retirement, after we no longer have to work so hard and save.

Imagine the frustration of knowing that you were dying! Would this not be unjust? Would you not wonder: Why me? Why now? Would you not be angry—with the doctor who does your yearly physicals and did not discover your disease in time, or with fate, or with God? And those loved ones—would you not be just as furious if your significant other was dying? Does this question help us to see the need for denial and anger? It is seldom the welcomed time!

For most people, the how and how not to die answer was

probably quickly, in my sleep, painlessly. But then we begin to realize the impact of this suddenness on loved ones. Also there would then be no opportunity for unfinished business, no time for I love you's, or I'm sorry's. Most people, however, would not choose a slow deterioration of the body or the mind either; and certainly not pain and suffering.

Most people want to spend the end of life at home in a familiar environment, where they are able to give up things at their own pace. People choose to have their friends and family gathered around, but would also want to be able to communicate with them. We would not want to be a burden to them. Therefore the requirements are: no pain, still mobile, still independent, with full intellectual abilities; but with a prognosis, a little time to put things in order. That, perhaps, would be the least worst way to die.

The answers to who goes first have to do with coping strengths. Who could handle the suffering and care of the other with less difficulty; who could manage the loss best? The hope is that at least one could survive the grief process and be able to go on with life. Much of our bereavement work must address these dependency problems, because, of course, the person who dies is not always the one whose loss the family can most easily survive.

For bereavement support, caregivers must know of many resources to help with financial and legal assistance; emotional problems; physical implications and handicaps; and the whole realm of resocialization and remotivation opportunities, such as senior centers, widow-to-widow groups, family counseling centers, volunteer and employment referral agencies, churches, etc.

What do we fear most? The fear of death itself is usually realized to be a fear of the unknown. For most people, it is the fear of dying that causes the most concern. People fear pain; isolation from loved ones; causing financial strain on the family; being an emotional burden for loved ones; being the cause of grief, immobility, dependency, personality change. Will I be able to handle the suffering? The physical deterioration? Will my mind go? Who will I be when I am dying? Will my religious beliefs hold up?

Many of our patients want to explore their spirituality. Whether they were deeply religious, somewhat interested, or not all religious during their lives, it often assumes immediate importance at the time of dying. In order to be able to support a person in their faith, we must have our religious house in order. For example, I am a Christian. I am also very busy. Therefore, I have learned that I must plan to allow myself the time for opportunities to strengthen and renew my faith, and then I am kept prepared to swing into a caregiving role. If we have our house in order, we neither have to defend nor sell our way. We will then be able to support people in their backgrounds and beliefs because we are free to accept it as their way.

The preceding exercise is an attempt to call attention to the problems and concerns of patients and families that derive from the four questions posed. Caregivers must be in touch with their own fears in order to be able to place themselves in a position of trying to understand what the other person is communicating.

Dealing with the reality of death is an ongoing process at Hospice. We have built into our program the opportunity to vent and share feelings. We not only listen to our patients and families, we also listen to each other. We expect our personnel to get involved with patients, and therefore we know that feelings about death and actual grieving over the loss of persons are going to continually recur.

We who are 40 years of age or older have probably been taught the importance of maintaining a professional detachment so as not to get sucked into another person's problems. The theory is that if you let a drowning man get his hands on you, you are both likely to go under. But the dying and grieving person needs someone with whom to share his suffering. We have learned how to enable our professionals and nonprofessionals to share suffering, to allow the dying and grieving to get their hands on us and to hang on tight. We do this by not allowing the the caregiver to be out in deep water alone and unprepared. We train our "lifeguards" well and try to make sure that they have ample recreation and refreshment time. But, most important, our team works like a long chain of caregivers holding hands, and we always make sure one is standing on the shore. When it looks like a patient is beginning to drag one of our team members under, the whole team pulls harder. When a team member is getting tired and has had enough, the colleague on the shore replaces him.

This is the essence of teamwork and team support. We feel it is essential for sustaining all caregivers. You must find someone with whom to share your load, if you wish to get involved with dying persons.

Think again of the answers to the when, how, who first, and fear most questions. The dying have much to teach us about living!

A dying person goes through a process of separation, beginning with the last important ideas, things, and people in his life, and then working slowly toward the center of his life, letting go in priorities of importance, with the last letting go being that group of people who are most special, and finally the most significant other person in his life.

With our questions, we were trying to conceptualize what it would be like to be dying. What if we were really given a prognosis of 3 months? What changes would we make in our life-style? With which people would we wish to be? How would we spend our time? Our patients and families teach us to live, to enjoy this precious gift of life.

Think for a moment of your past week. Sometime write down the way you spent your last 168 hours of life and see what changes you would plan for next week if it were one of your last. The urgencies and emergencies of this day become less important when we begin to set our priorities.

Do we rejoice in the wonder of a moment with a child? Will we experience the next glorious spring? Do we taste our food, walk in the woods, run in the surf, hear the birds, hug a friend, feel our healthy bodies? Do we explore the intricacies of our minds? Do we sing? Do we pray? One of my most enjoyable times is the moments I spend in a bathtub, with hot water up to my neck. I enjoy the warmth. I enjoy the solitude, that I am able to be there alone. I enjoy it because I know people who are unable to bathe themselves or even get into a tub.

By setting priorities we will become less the busy, harried, nervous clockwatchers. We will prioritize our work load to enable more minutes of direct caregiving. We will schedule times for recreation and refreshment. We will be better able to utilize our professional skills because we are refreshed and alive!

When I am dying, I will want to know that my caregivers have personal experience with all of the joys of life that I am losing, because then they will be better able to understand my suffering and better equipped to help!

Hospice was described as one of the units of support in the New Haven area. Then were listed the other units with whom we work in a cooperative and complementary system of support. This is the support system of coordinated small systems that dying patients need.

The physician. The dying patient needs a physician who remains primary physician, who continues to provide care when all attempts at cure have been exhausted, who has expertise in the management of pain and other symptoms such as vomiting and diarrhea caused by disease or the treatment of the disease, who cooperates with other disciplines to treat the social and psychological components of physcan pain, who makes home visits when needed.

The public health nurse. The dying need a public health nurse who teaches family members skills of making a bed with the patient in it; how to deal with incontinence; how to transfer the patient from bed to chair, prepare special diets, feed the patient, give and understand medication; and to be on call for home visits during the nights and weekends for emergency questions and treatment.

The acute care hospital. The dying need an acute care hospital that has personalized admitting and discharge procedures; space provision for families; flexible visiting hours; children allowed; procedures for allowing family members to continue to provide care; flexible meal hours and food selection; procedures for continuing comfort measures that were found effective at home such as special diets for bowel control, sherry for sleep.

The pharmacy.   The pharmacy must be one that provides 24-hour, 7-days-a-week availability of drugs and supplies that might be needed by a physician or nurse to provide precise symptom management in the home; and a 24-hour delivery service.

The social worker.   The dying patient needs the social worker who helps patients and families understand the effects that dying has on the family system, interprets these effects for personnel in other systems, provides advice and resources for financial and legal problem solution, and helps families identify and effectively utilize family strengths.

Service organizations.   Service organizations are needed to provide meals on wheels, transportation for clinic and physician appointments, medi-car and ambulance service, homemakers, childsitters, patient sitters, people to run errands and shop for supplies, laundry service, bereavement support groups.

Clergy.   The dying patient and his family need clergy who cooperate and communicate with the other discipline support systems, who make home visits, and who train and supervise support groups within churches and synagogues to provide pastoral care for the dying and grieving members of their congregation.

The circle of friends.   The dying need their circle of friends who express their grief; help with patient care; gather around the family to provide the emotional and practical support within the realm of their abilities, experience, and skills; who fill in the gaps and help in emergencies.

The people in the systems just described need to have an understanding of the problems and concerns of people who are experiencing the end of life; they need to develop active listening skills within the perspectives that have been discussed; they need to learn to work together to avoid duplication of services and to prevent fragmentation and confusion for families.

The Hospice program in New Haven is designed to supplement, not duplicate, the available services of the existing health care system. Hospice refers patients and families to all of the appropriate resources in the community and fills in the gaps with our personnel. We then assume the responsibility for communication between systems to improve the continuity of care and the coordination of services.

To continue to fill the needs for support that are communicated by patients and families, we must continually change and develop our programs as new needs are identified and as other systems change areas (or the quality) of their services. There is always much new work to be done in areas of interagency and interdisciplinary cooperation; and much new work to be done in education, not only for professionals, but for the public as well.

As institutions, agencies, private practice professionals, and nonprofessional organizations continue to develop mechanisms for cooperation and coordination of service for persons at the end phase of life, services will increase and improve. We have learned in New Haven that when most of the needs for help are heard and met with understanding, the processes of dying and grieving can be managed by the patient/family unit.

The family system is the appropriate and preferred support system for dying and grieving. Our task is to continue to learn from the dying what help is needed, and to be willing to change old systems and design new ones accordingly.

Chapter 6

PSYCHOTHERAPY
Bennett S. Gurian

Psychotherapy cannot be discussed in a vacuum. Reference must be made to what we do for people, to people, or with people in the context of some mutual understanding about the nature of normal aging and the nature of the pathology seen in aging, so that we can begin to address the therapeutic interventions that make sense for each entity.

When I was a fledgling psychiatrist in my first year of residency at the Massachusetts Mental Health Center and anxious about working with mentally ill people in the hospital, one of my professors at that time, with whom I shared my anxiety about sitting with these very difficult patients, said, "Don't worry, you're probably not going to do much harm." I gave up the rescue fantasy and the marvelous image of the physician who can heal and cure and change the course of peoples' lives long ago. I now have a much more restricted and limited goal as a therapist; one which involves more of a person-to-person than a doctor-patient kind of relationship.

Along those lines, I recently came upon some comments by Jerome Frank, professor emeritus of psychiatry at Baltimore. He was talking about a demoralization hypothesis, and he said, "Psychotherapy is a process whereby a socially sanctioned healer seeks to help persons overcome psychologically caused distress and disability, by a systematic procedure linked to a theory of the source and nature of the sufferer's difficulties and how to alleviate them."

That is an eloquent statement of the medical model, in which our approach is based on understanding the etiology of the pathological condition, coming up with a treatment plan that is rational, and then following it to conclusion, hopefully to improve or relieve the symptoms.

Historically, psychotherapy started as moral treatment; thus the etiology of the pathology—the source of the trouble—was seen to be demons. We then moved to a biophysical approach, wherein the origin of the disease process was seen to be bugs. We next moved to the psychoanalytic approach, in which the origin of all our troubles was seen to be intrapsychic. We now embrace the community mental health approach, wherein the source of all our troubles is seen to be "society"; i.e., the environment.

Therapy implies pathology; otherwise, there would be no need for therapy. What we have to learn much more about are the differences between a normal old person and a normal young person, a healthy old person and a healthy young person, before we can decide what the sicknesses of old persons are really about. There is a bona fide body of knowledge that does constitute a subdiscipline within psychiatry at this time: It has been called geriatric psychiatry. The term is about 5 years old. All my earlier papers referred to the field as psychogeriatrics, so here I am retracting. The term psychogeriatrics puts the emphasis on the medical aspects of mental illness in old age, while geriatric psychiatry puts the emphasis, just as in child psychiatry, on the underlying psychological dysfunction.

UNIQUE PROBLEMS PRESENTED BY THE ELDERLY PATIENT

When we look at older persons, we see certain diseases that primarily occur in the latter phase of life; this includes medical diseases as well as psychiatric illnesses. Some of the medical diseases are Parkinson's disease, the dementias, normal-pressure or low-pressure hydrocephalus, decubitus ulcers, accidental hypothermia, urinary incontinence, strokes, polymyalgia rheumatica, osteoporosis and osteoarthritis, carcinoma of the prostate gland, chronic lymphocytic leukemia, tuberculosis (especially miliary tuberculosis), varicella zoster (known as shingles), and probably basal-cell carcinoma of the skin.

Another way of looking at disease in old age is not which diseases commonly occur in old age, but what happens to a person who is older and develops a disease that someone at any age can get. The older person may respond differently.

Special problems attend someone who has thyroid disease in old age, for example, hyperthyroidism. It may present, in fact, in a masked fashion characterized by apathy, rather than the agitated hyperactivity of the hyperthyroid younger patient. Hypothyroidism in the elderly may present as a gradual decline and depression leading to nursing home care and death without ever having been diagnosed.

Pneumonia may occur in old age without fever. What is different about the older person who may have afebrile pneumonia, while the same virus in a younger patient will produce elevated temperature? I have seen pulmonary edema in older persons without shortness of breath; yet that symptom is one of the hallmarks of the disease. Silent carcinoma also occurs, especially of the bowel, lung, and sometimes the breast. Of older persons who have myocardial infarction, 20% do not report chest pains, and present instead with confusion and disorientation. Much later, when they have recovered, they may remember that they did have chest pain; yet the presenting symptom was not the usual left-sided pain.

Thus we know that there are some diseases and some ways

of responding to them among older people that do distinguish them from people of other ages. There is something special about being old.

All this does not mean that old people are sick; on the contrary, most old people are healthy. Most old people live in their own homes, in the community, and only 16% at any one moment in time have any major decrease in their usual level of activity. These are the vast majority of older persons, the ones we hear nothing about, the ones with whom we do not deal, the ones who are not referred to us. It is true that one third of them are living at the poverty level, which is not nice; they are unhappy and their quality of life is not necessarily good, but they are not sick.

The elderly also tend to deny real illness. We as caregivers suffer the same kind of prejudicial approach to old age as do the elderly. This was very interestingly demonstrated in the United Kingdom when Sir Ferguson Anderson, one of the greatest gerontologists of our time, did a study of a huge sample of elderly people living in the community and demonstrated very clearly that they do not seek medical attention even when they have acute illnesses such as fractured hips, pneumonias, and urinary tract infections. When doctors interviewed patients who had been identified as having a fractured hip, they would say, "That's just being old; I thought it was just because I was old." This is the same outworn mythology, that old means sick, and it is just not true.

ATROPHIC DISEASES OF THE CENTRAL NERVOUS SYSTEM

A controversy exists with respect to the atrophic diseases of the central nervous system (CNS), i.e., the loss of brain tissue resulting in either behavioral or personality changes or both. The controversy centers on whether cortical atrophic diseases should be included under the rubric of geriatric psychiatry, or is more appropriately contained within medicine and neurology. As a practicing clinician required to evaluate and treat either the person who comes to me or the person I go to, I have to know about both and take care of both; for functional disorders and atrophic CNS diseases very often present together.

I choose to include what has in the past been called organic brain syndrome as a valid part of my practice in geriatric psychiatry, and I teach that it should be included because (1) sometimes it is inseparable from a presentation of a functional disorder; (2) sometimes they present simultaneously; and (3) I take a holistic approach to the patient. A geriatric psychiatrist is well versed in internal medicine, and the internist, 80% of whose practice is psychosomatic medicine, ought to know something about psychiatry.

I am not comfortable using the term organic brain syndrome. One does not say organic foot syndrome or organic heart syndrome or organic left kidney syndrome. Not only the brain, but the central nervous system is involved. There is not just one syndrome; rather, the brain, as the most complicated mass of protoplasm in our body, has a few common pathways through which it can respond to a stress presented to it. You can kick this computer; or you can throw electricity through it, poison it, starve it, and it is going to show the effects with a certain few reactions, like memory loss, confusion, cognitive impairment.

How about the words chronic and acute? I don't like those either. The word chronic, for instance, by and large, implies therapeutic nihilism, which is dangerous. If we say something is chronic, we tend to think in terms of less active kinds of therapeutic approaches.

What is an "acute" brain syndrome? Somebody hit by a car may sustain head trauma, and thus have an acute brain syndrome. It is possible that it will worsen and remain a chronic problem. It may be acute in terms of time, but not in terms of remission or treatability.

We might better think in terms of the brain beginning to

manifest symptoms of underlying pathology in a number of different ways. One way is that the mass of functional brain has reached a critical point, a decrease in functional mass, where it can no longer provide us with its usual highly complicated sophisticated integrating circuitry. We thus lose some of our higher mental functions. They are our most recent acquisitions phylogenetically, and they seem to be the first to go. As we become more and more impaired, we are left with residual primitive functions of the central nervous system.

Another way of looking at it is according to Lashley's theory of mass action, proposed many decades ago, in which adjacent parts of the brain will pick up certain lost functions within certain limits. It has its own inherent intelligence. If a piece of it on one side is damaged, maybe an adjacent piece can do something about that. There is a limit to the degree of repair, governed by all kinds of anatomic and electrical boundaries. Past a certain point of disease or destruction of brain tissue, the brain cannot pick up and take over other parts of its own function, in which case one presents with symptoms, either behavioral or personality changes.

Differential Diagnosis
of Mental Illnesses in Later Life

It may be instructive to provide in a quick sketch an operational classification of the mental illnesses of later life. It is my attempt to synthesize three other major classifications: (1) the DSM 3; (2) the World Health Organization's monograph on psychogeriatrics; (3) the Busse and Pfeiffer book, *Mental Illness in Later Life.* I am not interested in all the fine points of nosology because, frankly, the only real advantage to classification is to help us as clinicians differentiate one disease entity from another, and they are not all that separate. Most of the patients with whom I have worked fall in between the cracks anyway. They have a little of this and a little of that.

Organic Disorders

One way of differentiating the brain diseases is to determine whether or not the origin (the source of the trouble), is within the bony calvarium or within some other part of the body. Thus, we call it either intracranial or extracranial. Intracranial causes can arise in any component within the bony calvarium. The brain itself is subject to primary neuronal degeneration. We call it primary neuronal degeneration because we do not know why it happens.

INTRACRANIAL ORIGINS. Those who work with older patients, especially in nursing homes, geriatric hospitals, or chronic disease hospitals have seen patients' records, that list cerebrovascular or arteriosclerotic vascular disease/senile dementia. About one third of patients coming to post mortem, who have manifested clinical symptoms of a true dementia during their lifetime, have in fact, some degree of arteriosclerosis in their cerebral arteries; but only about 10% of those are significant and can be correlated with a clinical state. Arteriosclerosis is a patchy disease occurring throughout the body; it is not systemic. A person whose brain has perfect patent arteries may have coronary arteries that are practically occluded.

Primary neuronal degeneration is the major cause of the clinical condition known as dementia. Other causes can involve diseases of the connective tissue that supports this gelatinous mass of brain cells; or of the cerebrospinal fluid that bathes the central nervous system; or of the bone itself that encompasses it and houses it in a fixed, nonexpandable container. Finally, the cause can be tumor from any of these underlying tissues, or metastatic disease.

EXTRACRANIAL ORIGINS. Those diseases that occur outside of the calvarium and impact on the central nervous system in such a way as to produce symptoms of dementia, constitute what may be called extracranial origins. They include anemias, mal-

malnutrition, electrolyte imbalance, urinary tract infections, upper respiratory infections, drug intoxication, tumors, kidney disease.

One may also think of these syndromes in terms of their rate of onset, their duration, and their degree of severity. We may speak about dementia as mild or early, moderate or middle, severe or late, and these are interchangeable terms. This is not merely academic. It is important to be able to differentiate an early or mild dementia (which triggers in our medical model thinking certain therapeutic approaches) from the more severe and less responsive types of illness.

In my experience, not all the dementias just defined include thought disorder. Thus senile dementia and senile psychosis are not synonymous.

"Nonorganic" or "Functional" Disorders.

The nonorganic or functional disorders include the neuroses, psychoses, personality disorders, and situational disturbances.

The psychoses, in geriatric psychiatry, include four major presentations of thought disorders: (1) schizophreniform diseases; (2) bipolar or manic-depressive illnesses; (3) psychotic depression; (4) the paranoid state.

The neuroses in geriatric psychiatry include three major presentations: (1) depression, (2) anxiety, and (3) hypochondriasis. I chose to include hypochondriasis as a separate entity, although you will find the symptom of somatization present in a lot of different diseases. People will focus on a part of their body as a symptom, as a way of letting you know they are hurting, because they are unable to deal with underlying conflicted material that is too painful and too threatening to confront. It is easier for them to talk about low back pain, stomach trouble, migraine headaches, or angina, than it is to talk about an unresolved painful conflict.

The biologic process of aging does not automatically resolve unresolved adolescent conflicts, nor does it change your character. Guilt is a major part of depression in younger people, but depression in geriatric psychiatry seems to be more closely associated with loss.

Turning our attention now to the psychoses, schizophrenia is not simply an acute psychotic reaction, but a lifelong disease. It is chronic and recurrent, and may wax and wane. I don't believe such a thing as late-onset schizophrenia exists, although late-manifesting symptoms used to be called paraphrenia. People probably have the underlying genetic predisposition, the family background, the stresses, whatever is involved in the production of this disease, all their lives. It may have been handled in different ways throughout their lifetime and may manifest itself more obviously later in life. But it probably does not happen suddenly.

The two major diagnostic elements of schizophrenia are: (1) It is primarily a thought disorder, with poor reality testing, hallucinations, delusions, and looseness of association; and (2) there is a lifelong history of difficulty in object relations and human interactions.

There is true or process schizophrenia; there is the schizoid personality in which there is no true thought disorder; and there are schizoaffective states, which are a sort of combination between thought disorder and affective disorder. These I refer to as the schizophreniform complex of diseases.

Bipolar depression or manic-depressive illness by definition simply cannot be a depression; otherwise it would be a psychotic depression. There must be a history of some cyclic phenomena, either of true mania or hypomania.

The last psychotic illness we will consider is the paranoid state. Paranoia is usually seen as a symptom, not as a disease. Paranoia is a symptom of any number of illnesses, e.g., schizophrenia, depression, etc. But in the elderly we may see a single delusional presentation that is both fixed and resistant. Every other sphere, every other intellectual function is intact, except that when the 63-year-old woman comes home from   work where she has been performing well for 20 years, she walks into her apartment, pulls down the shade, and puts a towel under the door so that the gases will not poison her. She wakes up the next morning, goes off to work, and again does everything perfectly.

But we must beware not to label everything that smacks of suspiciousness as paranoia, especially in the elderly. It may be good reality testing. As we know, the elderly are molested, deprived, rejected, abandoned, hurt—all the things that anyone would complain about. One must check their reality situation carefully before diagnosing them as paranoid. Their fears and suspicions may in fact be based on true threats.

There are two views of depression. I had a teacher in medical school who said, "All that wheezes is not asthma," and I think of depression in the same way. All that is sad, all that is tearful, all that is lonely, is not necessarily clinical depression. But there are two camps, and you must choose for yourself. There is the broad inclusive diagnosis or classification that places all sadness in a spectrum, a continuum. There is a second camp (to which I belong), which says, there is normal grieving, normal mourning, normal reaction to loss, normal sadness. And then there are reactions that are pathological. When these reactions significantly get in the way of our functioning, then they constitute the disease called depression. It has many different forms.

No matter which view you take, you have to look for underlying treatable causes, not the least of which is medication. The two major drug types we have learned may produce depression are the reserpine drugs and the oral contraceptives.

The depressive disorders probably account for about 50% of all mental illness over the age of 65. One group of depressions is related to the schizophreniform diseases. Another is related to bipolar, manic-depressive illness, one part of which is depression. A third category of depression is the unipolar variety.

Subcategories of unipolar depressions include: (1) endogenous, (2) chronic characterological, (3) agitated involutional, and (4) nonspecific. With the aid of a good history you should be able to ascribe the depression either to the schizophreniform, the bipolar, or the unipolar diseases. But history alone will not enable you to distinguish among the unipolar depressions. This requires looking at the signs and symptoms of the disease. The different signs and symptoms that will help classify the unipolar depressions are now described.

Characteristic of endogenous depression are psychic retardation, dull and fuzzy thinking, indecisiveness, loss of energy, fatigue, impaired vitality, decreased ambition, and anhedonia (the inability to enjoy or to get gratification out of either work or leisure activities). There may be some degree of agitation; sleep, appetite, and/or bowel disturbances; a sense of hopelessness and helplessness; demoralization; and serious suicidal thinking.

Two important things should be remembered about the endogenous depression. First, the patient may not look or feel sad, but if the other components are present, it is likely an endogenous depression. The second interesting thing about this disease is that it does not respond well to environmental alteration or to social or interpersonal therapeutic intervention. It does respond well to chemotherapy, however.

It is instructive to compare the signs and symptoms of endogenous depression with those of chronic characterological depression. The person suffering from this form has a lifelong history of presenting exaggerated symptoms to minor stresses; he has made a poor social adjustment, is weepy, seems preoccupied with losses, and feels cheated by everything in life. The sufferer is typically histrionic and emotionally labile. He is also an attention seeker; and in this illness suicidal ideation may be a part of the attention-seeking behavior, as well as irritability, pessimism, anger, self-pity, and manipulativeness. There is also a qualitative difference between these two depressions. The interesting thing about chronic characterological depression is that, unlike endogenous depression, it responds to drugs; but it is effectively treated by interpersonal psychotherapy and by environmental manipulation.

Agitated or involutional depression usually presents as a unipolar endogenous depression. With this disease you may observe pacing, hand wringing, skin pinching, nail biting, and hair pulling. All of these movements appear to be not functional but rather self-inflicted punishment. One often hears patients describing their feeling that their bodies are gradually decaying, piece by piece; that they are falling apart. Since this disease generally appears in late middle age to early old age, we call it involutional; but it could occur at any age.

The fourth category of depression is the situational or reactive form. This is an overwhelming reaction to prolonged stress, such as grief. The patient is unable to bear the pain and go on with his life.

THERAPEUTIC INTERVENTION

Organic Disorders

If a thorough, comprehensive, orthodox screening, evaluation, and diagnosis of each elderly patient is done, one may find an underlying cause and treat it, leading to relief of psychiatric symptoms. We find that one third of the patients who ordinarily would have been shipped out to the back wards of state hospitals as senile and demented really are victims of treatable, reversible, acute confusional syndromes.

For the remaining population there is little that can be done to change the course of this progressive loss of brain tissue. The CNS does not regenerate. Since it is not usually a vascular problem, there is really no way to produce changes that will affect the brain cells by increasing blood supply with vasodilators or anticoagulants. Dementia is usually not caused by a vascular problem, with one exception: An entity called multiple small infarcts may account for less than 10% of these illnesses.

Many approaches have been tried. Many years ago hypobaric oxygen chambers were tried. Dr. Jacobs at Columbia said, "If the brain cell needs oxygen to function, and if it's being deprived of oxygen, well, let's place this person into an oxygen chamber and let them breathe 100% oxygen for several minutes," etc. To the best of my knowledge, attempts at replication by other laboratories have not yielded results that would support the hypothesis that having somebody breathe oxygen will lead to sustained improvement in mental function. If one thinks of this atrophic brain as going to sleep and therefore presents it with CNS stimulants, not only does it not work, but it may kill the patient. At this time, there is no good evidence from controlled studies that vitamins do a thing to change the course of this illness.

All of this should not force us into a position of therapeutic nihilism. There are things that can and should be done. The goals of the therapist are (1) to rule out what is treatable; (2) to understand what the capacities, resources, and strengths of that individual and of the primary group surrounding that individual are; and then (3) to do everything possible to support and maximize the potential of that individual in that family so that they can function at the highest possible level. Attendant to many of these organic processes is an associated depression or anxiety state or agitation. If a person cannot remember whether or not he just had dinner, it is going to make him afraid and angry. And if that person is walking around unable to calculate and give the right change at the supermarket and cannot remember where he parked the car, he is going to become depressed and demoralized. These are issues that are amenable to therapeutic intervention.

"Nonorganic" or "Functional" Disorders

Remembering that (1) patients do "fall between the cracks"; (2) we do misdiagnose; and (3) it is difficult to differentiate pseudodementia (which is truly depression) from dementia —all of this confusion sometimes forces us to resort to treatment in order to diagnose. A trial-and-error approach is perfectly acceptable. Do not feel guilty. If you try something and it fails to help, try something else. That may be the only way you can differentiate between disease entities. In all cases, even though I have indicated that endogenous depression does not respond well, the first approach must be interpersonal communication: dynamic, insight-oriented psychotherapy. Only when you have ascertained that this approach is not appropriate can you in good conscience move on to some other treatment modality.

The nature of the therapeutic relationship may vary, depending on the intellectual and emotional capacities of the patient. A flexibility of goals is essential for the therapist, even within a specific therapeutic relationship. Striving for unreachable expectations can only lead to further demoralization. Set reasonably high goals, however. We should not enter a situation thinking there is not much that can be done.

The type of intervention need not be intensive, individual, one-to-one therapy. Those of us who have been working with the elderly have had very positive experiences with group therapy. In addition to the insight work that can take place, there are the positive components of socialization and mutual support.

As in the Hospice approach (see Chapter 5) one should not identify the individual qua patient, but rather identify the primary group, patient, and immediate others (those in meaningful relationships to that person), as the focus of therapeutic intervention. Those who surround the patient can be either supportive or critical of your therapeutic intervention, in which case they can sabotage it.

In psychotherapy with older persons it is alright to be active. It is okay to let them become a little dependent on you, especially in the beginning. It is okay to do some symbolic giving. During my training years, we often were advised not to infantilize, not to make the patient dependent, etc. I believe that; but I also know that an older person who has undergone so many losses and is feeling such an emptiness, needs to be filled, needs someone to lean on. It does not become addictive.

Doctor Alvin Goldfarb used to preach this all the time: "Let them lean on your shoulder a little bit. Don't get scared. It's going to help establish an initial contact, a trust."

Be there on time! Be there when you committed yourself to be there. Let them know you are really there for them. And symbolic giving means not only of yourself and your caring; many other things can also be given. Medication sometimes has more potency as a symbolic gift than for its chemical actions.

Finally, we need to understand our own prejudices, our own attitudes about aging, so that they do not prevent our establishing an optimal therapeutic alliance.

One form of psychotherapy that I find very useful with older persons is intermittent support. I present a case below in which an initial phase of intensive work was followed by an important ongoing, perhaps lifelong relationship. An elderly client needs to know that when things get stressful, when he feels depleted, when the next loss comes along—that there is a caring person nearby with whom he can re-establish contact simply by lifting the phone. Don't be too busy to see them.

Psychoanalysis is currently being used as a treatment modality with older persons. Freud said it couldn't be done: You reach 35 and you're over the hill; forget it, you're rigid, can't learn any more. It is just not true.

Therapeutic intervention can refer, in addition to the individual or group type of intervention, to structured supportive environments such as day treatment. It is important to consider day care, day treatment, socialization, rehabilitation programs, especially in terms of aftercare or primary prevention. It is difficult to identify persons who are at high risk, since we do not really know what the risk factors are. We have paid a lot of lip service to the idea of factors such as isolation leading to depression, but there is little evidence for it. It seems to make sense; we think that when one is alone, one is sad. But little hard data exist to support our prejudices about what leads to mental illness.

If you think you are dealing with a person who is beginning to be sick, early intervention probably makes sense. If you can identify symptoms early and intervene early, then you have some chance of keeping that disease process from snowballing.

Day treatment offers the advantage of keeping elderly persons at home with family, familiar furnishings, clothing, pets, neighbors—in short, their usual way of life. It is also like going off to work. You get up in the morning and go to your day treatment, and then you go home. It can also maintain the cohesiveness of the family because having the older person out of the home during the day can reduce the level of resentment towards that older person. The younger person, usually the daughter taking care of mother, can go to work; the household can be freed up for a few hours a day. Day treatment may eliminate the need for full-time care or hospitalization or at least delay the need for institutional care, while providing socialization, nutrition, and therapy. If hospitalization can be avoided, we are making progress toward undercutting the usual regression seen in persons who have to be institutionalized.

The history of psychiatry, like the history of any therapeutic modality, is that when something new appears, it is seen as the panacea and everybody is treated with it. When shock treatment was first discovered, everyone was entitled to be shocked. Then there was a hue and cry that we had no idea what we were doing, that we were destroying brain tissue; it was like kicking the computer; it was immoral. Then nobody received shock treatment. I think that now the pendulum has swung back to a more reasonable, rational middle area. Suppose you have made a very careful diagnosis (limited to depressions involving agitation, psychotic thinking, suicidal ideation), and there is neither time to develop a good therapeutic alliance with the patient or client, nor for the tricyclic antidepressants to be effective. Suppose further that the patient is refusing to eat and will die from dehydration or malnutrition in three or more days, or has more actively attempted suicide and is climbing the walls in pain. You owe it to such a patient, and to his family, to try shock treatment. It should be done unilaterally, with an anesthesiologist in attendance. There should be no observable convulsive activity, except perhaps a flick of the toe to confirm that you have produced seizure activity, but not to the point where fracture is a danger, even in an osteoporotic patient. The only contraindications in the literature are a space-occupying lesion of the central nervous system or a recent or acute myocardial infarction.

Since psychotherapy often is more effective with adjunctive chemotherapy, the next area for consideration is the use of drugs.

1. Think of drugs last. The elderly are hoarders and guilty of polypharmacy. In their homes can often be found dozens of envelopes, boxes: perhaps medicine for the dog; something used by a spouse before death; or a plastic bag left by a neighbor on the doorstep. Few people, let alone the elderly, understand side effects or drug interaction. One of the major causes of confusional states, delirium, and death among the elderly is drug toxicity.

2. The aging body has an altered anatomy and physiology, so that no matter what the route of administration, the drug is neither absorbed, assimilated, metabolized, detoxified, nor excreted according to the nice curves in your pharmacology textbook. With drug therapy you risk producing toxic intermediary metabolites, unwanted drug interactions, and high tissue concentrations due to inadequate excretion, among other problems.

3. Elderly persons for whom you are prescribing drugs may have some degree of confusion and may therefore require constant supervision. Simply writing a prescription for somebody and saying, "Go home and take this," is asking for trouble. It is important that

somebody in the family, a neighbor, visiting nurse, or yourself, pay very close attention to the drug taking of an older person living in the community. A very high proportion (96%) of our older population live in the community, and this underscores the extent of our responsibilities.

4. Chemotherapy is very expensive. Since the elderly are the poorest minority group in this country, and are gradually becoming the poorest majority group in the country, they cannot afford expensive medication; neither are they reimbursed (under most plans) for such expenditures.

5. The aging usually are already taking at least three or four essential medicines, such as the heart pill, something to reduce blood pressure, probably something to assist in digestion or bowel excretion, maybe something for sleep, for diabetes—and probably something for arthritis. If you give psychoactive medication in addition to these essential drugs, you can imagine what is happening to that poor person's system.

6. The elderly may have idiosyncratic reactions to medications, some of them paradoxical. I have seen agitated older person treated with a barbiturate (a sedative hypnotic); instead of reducing the agitation, the barbiturates had the person climbing the walls. Stopping the barbiturates calmed the person considerably.

7. As a therapist, I think that my profession is guilty of the major abuse of putting medicine between us and our patients, just as the surgeon puts the mask on. It forms a barrier between us, because we are afraid and frustrated at not getting the immediate gratification of a cure; and possibly because we are anxious about our own old age or are identifying the patient with our own parents or grandparents. At any rate, we do feel pressured, not only within ourselves, but by the fami-

lies or the nursing home or the ward director of nursing: "You've got to do something; they're screaming all night," or "They won't take their medicine," or "They're having fights all the time with the staff." "Do something, doctor." We respond to the family. We respond to the inner voice telling us we must be helpers. We respond to the staff of the nursing home. And we practice bad medicine. We prescribe when we shouldn't prescribe.

These are the reasons I recommend that we think of drugs last. If you finally arrive at the conclusion that you have to use a medication, or in some instances that it really is the treatment of choice, then here are some rules of thumb:

1. Start small.
2. Build gradually.
3. Use as little as half the usual adult dosage.
4. When discontinuing a medication, decrease slowly.
5. Whenever you give a medicine to an older person, do your baseline vital sign examinations (blood pressure, respiration, pulse); and then do it periodically, especially soon after you start the medication, and watch for side effects.

Drug therapies may be associated with psychotherapies in the classifications discussed earlier.

With depressions, the CNS stimulants do not work, since they do not treat the underlying cause. In fact they may precipitate heart attacks, convulsions, agitation, increased respiration. We know that certain kinds of depressions seem to be associated with abnormal levels of circulating catecholamines. Monoamine oxidase (MAO) inhibiting agents are often good antidepressants. They work, but they are also capable of precipitating an acute hypertensive episode, i.e., a sudden abrupt increase in blood pressure, which in turn can precipitate a stroke. This may happen when the MAO inhibitors mix in the body with certain types of chemicals present in food stuffs that have been aged, such as certain cheeses and wines, nuts, and chocolate. Unless the person is in a hospital setting so that the diet can be knowledgeably supervised, it is not safe to prescribe the MAO inhibitors.

If you use neither the stimulants nor the MAO inhibitors, what are you left with to treat the depressions? The tricyclic antidepressants are the drugs most often used. A number of problems have been associated with the tricyclic antidepressants. They produce atropinelike effects, such as drying of the mucous membranes and bladder and bowel atony resulting in bladder distension, impaction, etc. They can precipitate psychosis. The major problem is in the cardiovascular system, however: The tricyclics produce what is called orthostatic hypotension. The blood pressure drops when the person sits up or stands up; this may lead to fainting, falling, head injuries, and even death. These drugs may also produce cardiac arrhythmias by causing electrical conduction problems in the heart.

The schizophreniform diseases (the psychoses) are best treated with a major tranquilizer. Again, psychotherapy and human interaction first; but, if you are also going to use drugs, use the major tranquilizers. The major tranquilizers also present a number of associated problems. Side effects include postural hypotension, sedation, and the production of a parkinsonianlike syndrome.

If you treat somebody who is psychotic with antipsychotic drugs, you may find him becoming progressively depressed. The psychosis itself may have been serving to protect the patient from confronting the underlying depression, and as you reduce the psychosis you then see the underlying depression. That patient may then become suicidal. The pacing stops, the hallucinations stop; but he wants to kill himself. We must be watchful and cautious. In manic-depressive illness, lithium carbonate should be started and used when the patient presents in a manic state. It has not proved effective if the patient is in the depressed stage of manic-depressive illness. However, once started on lithium and followed carefully with blood level determinations, the patient will probably have to be maintained on lithium for life. If depression appears you may have to add a tricyclic antidepressant. If a manic-depressive illness presents as an endogenous depression, you may have to start with a tricyclic antidepressant; when that begins to make them hypomanic then you start the lithium. The process of treating a manic-depressive patient, in addition to psychotherapy and intermittent support, is this juggling act of titrating the medication.

With the endogenous depressions, the tricyclics are the medication of choice. If one type fails, feel comfortable in trying the next one. We do not know a priori that they are all the same in terms of their therapeutic effectiveness.

A word about hypochrondriasis is in order, whether it stands alone or as part of another disease, as a somatization. Avoid becoming one of the "enemy out there" by telling the patient that it is all in his head. If you want to establish a therapeutic alliance, your approach has to be, "I hear you. It hurts, but instead of focusing on your back, let's talk about where it hurts inside. Is it your heart that's breaking? Let's get to the real issue. I hear you. I'm not putting you down. I believe you feel that pain."

The first draft of a case report I am writing may help to illustrate some of the points I have been trying to make here. This is an actual case from my own private practice. (I see elderly people in my private practice but not exclusively.) There are 75,000 practicing psychiatrists in this country at this time, but only 2% of us see patients over 65 in our private practice.

Mrs. R., 76 years old, was referred to me by her internist because of depression, suicidal thoughts, and an overwhelming concern about her 80-year-old husband's deteriorating mental status. She described herself as physically and mentally exhausted. I saw her in evaluation twice by herself and once with her husband in my office. She presented as an angry, bitter, frustrated woman who felt she had made a mess of her life by allowing herself to be "treated like a doormat" by her husband. Her mental status exam showed no evidence of cognitive impairment. Although Mrs. R. complained constantly, she resisted all efforts by her internist to help her elect options that might diminish her pain. She suffered from chronic obstructive pulmonary disease, and yet she continued to smoke two packs of cigarettes a day. She raged at the destructiveness and filth of their dog in the house, but would not agree to any of the suggested methods for getting rid of the dog. She was continually embarrassed, worried, and subject to significant financial loss through Mr. R.'s progressive dementia, but she would not proceed with the steps necessary to become his conservator or guardian.

Her medical history included neuromuscular hyperirritability, polycythemia, a 20-pound weight loss over a 3-month period, gradual hearing loss, hyperglycemia, and atrophic inflammatory vaginitis.

When I saw the couple together, their basic style of relating to each other was to make unilateral decisions without discussion between them; outrage and resentment then would bubble up between them, both in their home life and in their business life. Mr. R. had founded and was still active as the president of a large manufacturing firm, and Mrs. R. continued to function as the head of the advertising division of that firm. Their factory was about 600 miles away from their present home in Cambridge, Mass., and they both did extensive traveling back and forth to this business. They had not had sexual relations in 14 years, and they slept in separate bedrooms because she said he snored too loudly.

She stated that her overriding wish was to be taken care of by her husband, but instead his mental incompetence forced her into a position of accepting even more responsibility at this late point in her life. She had no family and no friends. The decline of her husband's health implied his impending death, which caused her more anxiety and anger toward him. She had spent recent months going from doctor to doctor, as if in an attempt to gather people who would care for her and fill the emptiness in her life.

Mr. R. was well-dressed and alert; his gait was normal, his speech clear, and he was somewhat suspicious. He blamed all this recent fuss on his wife's sudden and unexplained change in behavior. On mental status exam he showed significant impairment of intellectual function; he said that it was because he was not prepared for the test I was giving him, and that I was trying to trick him. By history, his confusion, memory loss, and poor judgment had progressed over the last several years.

My impression was that Mrs. R. suffered with both anxiety and depression, accentuated by facing a late-life crisis and compounded by a variety of uncomfortable somatic problems. We agreed to meet together twice each week for several weeks with the goal of helping her recognize and accept her husband's progressive impairment so that she could begin to alter her expectations from him and learn where she was waging an irrational battle; this would allow her to let go of her self-destructive components. With the help of her internist, we would evaluate further the possibility of using psychoactive medication. That was our contract.

I also agreed to see them as a couple whenever it seemed reasonable and offered to take legal responsibility for designating Mr. R. as mentally incompetent, if and when she felt able to apply for conservator or guardianship.

I worked with her and them for 18 months. The following issues are representative of the course of her therapy.

We met twice a week for the first several weeks, then once a week for several months. After 1 year, we began meeting once a month. She had come to me from her internist on Valium (diazepam) for the neuromuscular irritability, 10 mg at night. I changed the dosage pattern to 5 mg in the morning and 5 mg at night. Thus she got the same overall 24-hour dosage, but was taking something twice instead of only once. I added, with consultation from the internist, small amounts of Elavil (amitriptyline) 10 mg bid, and increased the dosage gradually until she was taking 75 mg/day. She remained at that dosage for 3 months until we had a firm working alliance, and she was feeling less depressed; at that point I lowered the dosage to 25 mg at bedtime, where it remained at termination.

Mrs. R. disclosed a suicide plan based on a newspaper article entitled "Pain Reliever Peril," which told of the potential danger of taking Darvon (propoxyphene) and alcohol together. She disposed of her Darvon, gave me the article, and told me she had decided that because of her vanity she could not take her own life, that it would be admitting to total failure.

Our sessions usually began with Mrs. R. in tears, shaking, and stating she could not go on. I encouraged a limited amount of dependency during this initial phase of our work and at the same time noted her many strengths and commented on them in simple descriptive fashion. She phoned me frequently during the first 6 months, and I encouraged her to do so. It was usually to tell me that she felt she could not go on, and as soon as I had arranged an extra or an earlier appointment with her, she would begin to apologize for taking so much of my time. She would then calm down and thank me for believing in her.

As she began to explore her options regarding the business, she expressed her concerns about being both elderly and a woman. She told me she had read about a Mrs. Knox, who when widowed at the age of 75, found herself heiress to the Knox gelatin company and spent the next 8 or 10 years of her life building and expanding the business. It was important for Mrs. R. to know that her situation had been faced by other elderly women, and she found comfort and reassurance in realizing that the challenge could be met and that there existed role models with whom she could identify.

During this phase of our work she told me of two dreams she had had repeatedly during the preceding year. In the first she was trying to jam more items into her suitcase than it could hold. In the second she was running after a train and missed it. She was able to see that both reflected the anxiety and the frustration attendant to her sense of inadequacy.

Her ambivalence regarding assuming guardianship for her husband was resolved in a complicated way. On a physical examination, Mr. R. was found to have bilateral inguinal hernias and was admitted to hospital for surgery. He was discharged from hospital to a nursing home, very confused and uncooperative. The internist then signed the papers, and Mrs. R. finally had her lawyer arrange for her to become his guardian at the nursing home. (I had made two home visits to them during the year prior to this incident, and I had signed those same papers twice. But each time she had refused to go ahead and take the legal action. She was not ready for it.)

At this writing, 2 years after we began therapy, Mrs. R. is no longer suicidal, her weight has stabilized, she has guardianship for her husband. She is now the director of the manufacturing firm and is having a private outside audit made in preparation for either consolidation or a potential sale of the business. She is taking no antidepressants, and we have terminated treatment with the understanding that she will call me whenever she wants to.

The points I have tried to make in this case presentation are (1) you do not treat an old person as an old person, you treat them as a person; (2) you deal with your own prejudicial views of what a "nice" old woman ought or ought not to do; and (3) you need to find out what she wants for herself and support her in doing that.

I encouraged some dependency early on. I gave symbolically; medication as well as time and permission for phone calls. She became neither unreasonable nor infantile. She went on toward independence and strength while still struggling with childhood fantasies and wishes to be cared for, to be dependent, and to have the man in charge. She worked those issues through at age 78.

Chapter 7

ATTITUDES AND AGING: US/USSR CONTRASTED*
Gari Lesnoff-Caravaglia

The Soviet Union, in the eyes of its people, is a developing or emerging nation. Past history is largely discounted, and the Soviets look upon their current state as having been born out of the 1917 Revolution and as being only some 60 years of age.

As a newly emerging nation, the Soviets feel that many of the problems that beset their country are due primarily to this condition. Soviets make constant reference to the fact that things are better than they were, and that they will improve even more in the future. Frequently reiterated phrases are: Things may still be far from satisfactory, but they are much better than they were 10 years—or 15 years—ago.

Unfortunately many Soviets have no way of comparing their current or past situation with living or working conditions in other nations. A trip like that of a few hours by air from

*Research sponsored by the Fogarty International Center under the US/USSR Agreement for Technical and Scientific Cooperation.

Moscow to Copenhagen presents striking contrasts and is more like crossing from one planet to another.

Out of this framework have developed the Soviet attitudes toward aging and older persons. The older generation is regarded as having participated in another culture—and is thereby a disadvantaged group.

Attitudes in themselves are complex areas for study. How they develop, why they develop, and what factors have contributed to their formulization are problems difficult to decipher. Yet these very complex conceptualizations, deeply embedded as they are in the cultural framework, affect behaviors in a very profound sense. Attitudes toward older persons are deeply rooted in cultural norms and expectations, and reflect fundamental responses to life itself.

For this reason, any analysis of attitude must take into consideration the societal milieu, along with current problem areas that impinge on the particular group under study. It was for this reason that the word compare was not chosen for the title, but rather contrast; for in some sense, cultures defy comparison and can only be studied through contrast.

In the main, three areas will be considered as they relate to older persons: the family, the economic situation, and health care. Naturally, there will be some overlapping within these topics. Contrasting examples from the United States will not be deliberately alluded to, but the focus will be placed upon those conditions that provide the greatest contrast.

The Soviet Union covers a wide geographic area, and has some 250 million inhabitants, 11.8% of whom are age 60 and over. In the Soviet Union statistics regarding older persons begin at age 60, as the retirement age is 60 for men and 55 for women. There exist a number of variations in retirement age; these are related to the job profile or the kind of work activity in which the individual is engaged.

Although the Soviet Union regards itself as an emerging nation, this does not mean that all vestiges of the old culture have totally disappeared. Many aspects of the old culture have been redefined and sometimes reshaped to meet particular current needs and interest. Some features of Soviet life bear strong resemblance to the past—in positive as well as negative instances.

A plurality of cultures is much in evidence in the 15 Soviet republics, which are regarded as unique entitites in much the same way as are the states within the United States. In some of these republics, a totally different language is spoken, with the Russian language appearing as the official or second language. One such example is Soviet Georgia. The majority of the people speak in Georgian, while most have a knowledge of Russian, particularly the younger generations. The elderly—those in the category of the long-living and those living in principally rural areas—in many instances neither understand nor speak Russian, and Soviet gerontologists must make use of interpreters in communicating with them.

The Soviet Union has long made use of a series of age classifications in studying the elderly population; this we find recent reference to in American literature. In the Soviet Union the categorization is as follows:

Zrosli (mature): 60–75 years

Starii (old): 75–90 years

Dolgozichili (long-living): 90+ years

In the United States the categorization is as follows:

Young Old: 60–75 years

Old Old: 75+ years

Because of the wide diversity of cultures within the Soviet Union, only two cultures will be described: the Russian, which is found primarily in the western north-central portion of the nation; and the Georgian, which is located in the southern portion.

Because of the diversity found in the Soviet republics, which is also present in the United States but to a much smaller degree, one must understand that exceptions can be found to some of the generalized statements to follow.

THE FAMILY

The family in the Soviet Union, like the American family, is by and large small in size. The average family includes one or two children; most families have only one child. Families of three or four children are considered large. The response to the question whether there were many families with as many as eight children was outright laughter, with the comment that that would be exhibiting poor common sense in light of current living conditions. The small family size is due primarily to the work style of family members, housing shortages, the materialistic ambitions of the family, and the absence of religious strictures related to birth control. Even the traditional religious position permitted birth control, abortion, and divorce.

Although the primary family unit is small, the relationship between generations and the extended family of cousins, aunts, and uncles is a very close one. Not only do family members see a great deal of one another; but when the opportunity arises, albeit rarely, to relocate to another area, many persons forego the opportunity because they prefer to remain close to relatives. The affection and respect shown the grandparents is part of this general family closeness.

The presence of the grandmother or grandfather in the home of a young family is not at all unusual. The role of the grandmother, or babushka, has become something of a national institution. The grandfather, or jedushka, sometimes plays a parallel role, but only in rare instances, for Soviet men retire later, often continue in gainful employment following retirement, and have a shorter life expectancy.

Even where there are state-supported nursing homes or homes for the elderly available, older family members are not generally placed in them. Approximately 200,000 (.5%) older persons reside in institutional settings. This is in sharp contrast to the American current, however debatable, 5% to 6%.

The respect and reverence for the elderly is deeply rooted in the old Russian tradition and religion, in the non-Russian republics such as Georgia as well. The presence of the babushka in the home results from several factors: the expectation that one takes care of one's own aging family members, coupled with the reverence for the aged.

As illustration, the director of the Ministry of Social Welfare in Georgia, who when interviewed was responsible for homes for the elderly and home health care for older persons, had a mother 97 years old. Her mother for the past 10 years had been bedfast and suffering from a debilitating illness that required 24-hour nursing care. The director, her sister, and a brother were working in shifts around the clock to care for their mother. They had been doing this for 10 years, and the director said that their mother would continue to receive such care until the moment of death. This woman, as director of the Ministry of Social Welfare, could easily have placed her mother in the best nursing home and could have commanded for her the best of care. To the director, this was unthinkable as long as there was a family to provide such care.

An additional factor allowing family members to be kept at home is that physicians make house calls. Not only are the services of a physician available in terms of home health care, but a visiting nurse, social worker, and a variety of community services are also available in some locations.

The presence of the babushka has also other important bearings on family life. She is *the* baby-sitter, as there is almost no domestic help for hire. With an older family member in the home, the mother is free to continue her employment or her career training without interruption. Care of the children, responsibility for the daily shopping (which means standing for hours in line for each commodity you might wish to purchase), and general housekeeping are often tasks assumed by the babushka and are regarded as acceptable ways of relating to the family of her child (usually a daughter). The daughter will, in most instances, take responsibility for the preparation of the evening meal, while the husband helps the child with homework if he/she is of school age.

The babushka may move in with the family or not, as she prefers. It is to the family's advantage to have her move in with them for a number of reasons. All of the grandmothers receive a pension; most of them, if not all, have worked. This pension, plus free public medical care, makes the babushka independent of the family in financial terms. In fact, many grandparents provide financial assistance to their mature children.

Some grandmothers prefer to continue working after reaching the age of 55. They may also prefer to maintain their own apartments. This choice is also accepted as proper, and, although the children may wish their parent had decided otherwise, this does not affect the closeness of the relationship. Young couples speak with something bordering on envy of friends who do have their babushka living with them. Such a decision to live independently is not necessarily on the rise since women in the Soviet Union have had the opportunity to follow careers since the 1920s.

Recognizing this new direction, however, the national government will soon permit women to remain at home from work after the birth of a child until the child is a year old—on full salary. There are also state nurseries that care for young children (yasli).

A great deal of pride is taken in the children by all family members. Although consumer goods, clothing in particular, are very hard to come by, the children are usually well dressed. At times the only color on the drab Soviet streets is the gaily colored clothing of a passing child.

Thus it is not at all unusual for three generations to be living together. Even after the children are grown, they may live at home while attending an institute. The student receives a stipend (average 50 rubles a month); which is more than adequate for a single person to live on and will also contribute to the family income. The son or daughter will live at home until he/she marries. Because of the pension and student stipend system and the fact that everyone is either working or going to school, no adult family member is financially dependent upon another. Much of the family strife related to money problems in American families simply does not exist in the Soviet Union.

The director of the Institute for Advanced Training of Physicians in Leningrad spent considerable time describing to this writer the beautiful relationship between his mother, who lived with his family, and his grown son. He described with great affection the way the grandson would keep his grandmother supplied with choice little tidbits at the breakfast table, and how he would encourage her to eat. This grandmother also brought with her all of her religious icons when she moved in with her son.

The presence of the grandmother in the home has other benefits. The allocation of apartments (and most urban populations live in apartments) is based on number of square meters per person. Accepting the grandmother in the home means that the family can apply for a larger apartment. The grandmother, in effect, has a right to a room of her own. Of course, it is not unusual for the beloved grandchild to share that room.

The benefits to the grandmother are also great. She has a meaningful role to play within the family and society. She is really needed. She lives within the warmth of the family environment. Her needs are met; she is usually respected by her son-in-law and adored by the children, whom she spoils.

I met one such babushka on the plane from Leningrad to Tblissi, the capital of Soviet Georgia. She had been visiting one daughter, and was on her way home to Tblissi, where she lived with a second daughter. She told me how she had raised one of her grandsons who lived in Leningrad, from the time he was several months old until he reached high school age. He was a model student, and as she said, "What can I say when the boy states openly that he loves *me* the best?" The bringing up of this grandson gave her a great deal of satisfaction. This babushka was 70 years old. As we started our downward descent, she kept craning her neck toward the windows; and then finally, in the manner of all Russians, speaking aloud as though there were no one around to hear, she said, "They both came. The darlings!" Both daughter and son-in-law were standing outside the reception area facing the airfield. The grandmother literally beamed.

There is great genuine attachment to aging parents. Part of this is also related to the suffering the elderly parents had endured in terms of their historical past.

As part of the history they are taught, children learn to identify their obligations as citizens as properly directed toward the elderly. The flowers they are taught to bring to the hospitals, the visits they make to the elderly living alone, and the organized helping groups developed through youth organizations such as the Young Pioneers, all serve to promote the well-being of the deserving elderly; they also introduce the children of increasingly small families to members of other generations.

In the family life of the long-living in Georgia, moderation in all things is stressed; this is actually a religious orientation. They are tranquil, gentle people, for the most part, and their being described as the Sicilian element in the Soviet Union can only be partially substantiated.

Within this congenial family life, no one ever shouts or raises his/her voice; no one scolds or belittles the children. Many have had relatives who were long-lived, and such long life is ascribed by Soviet gerontologists as due primarily to genetic factors. The long-living Georgians openly enjoy life, their work, and their families. A gentleman of 97 interviewed in the city of Tblissi gave a long and detailed account of his life, which reflected many of these features.

The Georgians do not retire because they believe that being actively engaged in work promotes well-being and good health. Once they become ill or physically incapable of work, they seem to gradually shrivel up and die. After the age of 120, they seem to shrink and then die of old age. One could ascribe a particular illness to the death, but (and these were physicians speaking) it is best described as death due to old age. The organism gradually weakens, and they die in bed or sitting in a chair.

Such advanced age has received documentation through birth certificates (the Soviet Union has kept such records for the past 150 years), the recall of past events, birth dates of children, date of marriage, or the date of parents' deaths, which can be authenticated on tombstones. The oldest person on record was a man of 168, who died several years ago.

Two thirds of the long-living are women, but the longest living are men. Women live an average of 8 years longer than do the men. Soviet Georgia is predominantly a male-dominated society. It is acceptable for a man of 90 to marry a woman of 40. Women at advanced ages do not marry, but occasionally a woman of 55 will bear a child. She is much embarrassed by this and tries to hide her condition.

Marriages of men at advanced ages, although they do occur, are rare. One man of 92 married a woman of 40; after 2 years of marriage, he could not understand why his wife had not conceived. Another example of a late marriage was a man of 72 who was married to a woman in her 30s: She bore him six children.

Soviet gerontologists accept the age of 120 as being commonly reached; there are some 5,000 long-living persons in Georgia; 72.5% of all the long-living in the Soviet Union are found in Georgia. There are 1,114 persons aged 100+ in the city of Tblissi, which has a population of 1 million.

Soviet gerontologists seriously question the advanced ages quoted by some of the long-living, and frequently relate jokes and stories with respect to such boasting. One doctor visiting the long-living in a village in Georgia spent some time talking with one gentleman; of course, he asked him his age. The man replied that he was 106. When the same physician was back in this village 6 months later, he again encountered the old gentleman, who remembered the physician. Again they enjoyed a long conversation, during which the physician asked once more how old the man was. This time the man replied 110. After a moment the old man turned to the physician and asked him why he looked so downcast, and the physician replied, "I am *so* sorry to hear that you have *aged* so much in just 6 months!" At this, the old gentleman laughed.

The stories as to the Georgian male's prolonged virility are also open to question. One man went to the doctor complaining that he was impotent. The doctor asked him his age, and the man replied 79. The doctor then said that at his age that condition was common. "But," the man protested, "my neighbor who is 81 keeps saying that he is still a 'whole' man."

"Well, then," replied the doctor, "you go home and do the same."

In discussing the long-living, Dr. G. Z. Pitzkalauri, Director of the Gerontology Center at Tblissi, commented that it is not those who utilized their mental capacities who live a healthy long life, but rather those who did heavy physical work. He stressed the importance of physical activity in prolonging life.

His studies had also indicated that bearing many children was conducive to longevity. This does not mean abortions, but children brought to term.

Actually, there are fewer long-living people in Abhasia near the Black Sea in spite of its fame. Abhasia has received "star" status because it has been frequently reported on, lies within a popular resort area, and is a convenient and pleasing place for reporters to spend some time.

THE ECONOMIC SITUATION

The retirement ages for men and women differ, with women retiring at age 55 and men at 60. There is also a difference in retirement age based on the type of work performed by the individual. In fact, a specialized branch of gerontology, gero-hygiene, has this as its primary interest. Every effort is made to describe each type of work according to its biophysiological demands upon the person.

Where such demands are great (in steel mills, for example), the retirement age is graded downward. A person could easily retire at 40 from one job, be assigned to another that is less physically demanding, and at 62 be reassigned to yet a third. His/her pension for the first job, however, continues in effect, and he/she can claim the regular salary for each subsequent position.

About 50% of the veteran workers—not retirees—continue working past age 55 or 60. Those who do not give as their reasons poor health, feeling that they had done their duty toward the state, or a wish to remain at home to help their children. This last reason is most frequently given by women, although it is not unusual to see the grandfather wheeling the baby carriage in the park.

Many of the problems older persons face are the same as those faced by the general population: shortage of housing; lack of consumer goods; food shortages; drab, routine existences; dictates from an ubiquitous authority; inability to relocate at will; and a general low standard of living. Thus the elderly are not singled out as a particularly deprived group; rather they participate in society on a par with the rest of the citizens.

Interestingly enough, in a recent study conducted by Dr. Nina Sachuk of the Kiev Gerontology Institute, one finding was that, although there did exist a flexible retirement system in the Soviet Union, persons facing retirement reported feelings of anxiety.

HEALTH CARE

Because of the cultural climate, in which psychosocial problems of the elderly do not loom large above those of other age groups, the major interest of Soviet gerontology has been biomedical in nature. Such an emphasis has led to the development of complexes such as the Kiev Gerontology Institute, which is made up of laboratories, outpatient and inpatient clinics, a center for the study of the long-living, an academic component; and there are plans for the development of a rehabilitation center.

Public health planning is an inseparable component of national economic planning. As a result, demography is an important aspect of health care, and is an important unit in every department of government. Since health planning involves the total nation, budgeting, allocation of personnel, distribution of services, and so on, must all be strictly carried out according to needs and numbers. Who the elderly are, what are their numbers, where they are to be found, and what are their health conditions, are vital information for such planning.

The organization of health care for the elderly is developed as a component within the general system of therapeutic and prophylactic health services serving the total population, and thus special mention of geriatric needs is not frequently made. There is great emphasis placed upon the accessibility of such services to all older persons, since the elderly constitute an increasingly large portion of the Soviet population and figure prominently in the work force.

The interest of the Soviet Union in keeping Soviet citizens as healthy and active as long as possible is, of course, linked to economic need. Also, one of the primary interests in studying the long-living is to gain resolution of some of the biomedical questions posed when persons live to advanced ages while suffering many of the same pathologies of which other people expire at younger ages. By extending the working life of the populace, the nation will be able to meet its economic demands more easily. This is particularly crucial in light of the decreasing birth rate.

The emphasis on preventive medicine in the Soviet Union derives from the same need. It is cheaper to keep people healthy, and to properly intervene, then it is to try to cure them of an ailment. The pre- and postnatal care, the special leaves for pregnant women, the emphasis on child medical care and treatment, are all predicated upon the need to develop a healthy and not only long-living, but long-productive people.

Since there is one physician for approximately every 320 residents (in what is termed a region), medical care is readily available for all persons regardless of age. In fact, because the physician treats persons of all ages, he/she develops the kind of practical expertise in dealing with the elderly that is only artificially imposed in rare medical training institutions in the United States.

The Soviet physician, since he/she works directly in the community, is in contact with many older persons who are productive community members. Many of the older persons are actively assisting in the welfare of their families, such as the babushka who cares for her grandchildren or the pensioner who has accepted a second lighter job that he continues until late in life. The physician thus does not have a stereotyped view of older persons, but his/her view of older persons is as varied as are impressions of any other age group.

Since medical care is free, the older person does not fear not having enough money to pay for medical care, nor is there the fear of living alone, for the justly famed emergency medical service (the "Skoraya pomosch") operates 24 hours a day. A citizen dials 03 on any phone, which connects him/her immediately with the operators of a central dispatching office. A crew of switchboard operators handles the incoming calls, referring those calls requesting judgmental decisions to the two physicians on duty. The physicians determine disposition of the problem and write the order; the dispatching switchboard crew then makes disposition—either by phone to its own ambulance station at the Center, or to one of 22 substations (in Moscow), or by radiophone to an ambulance already known to be in the area.

Each of these ambulances is manned by a medical staff that always includes a doctor, a driver, and at least one specifically trained feldsher (who approximates the American paramedical). The ambulances are specialized into coronary-care units, shock units, stroke units, and children's care ambulances; they are equipped and staffed accordingly.

While women account for over 90% of all feldshers in the Soviet Union, and 75% of all physicians, only 60% of the Skoraya feldshers are women because of the demands of this kind of work.

In at least two ways—by receiving a pension adequate for his/her needs and free medical care—the older Soviet citizen is free of the two primary fears that haunt older persons in the United States.

Older persons who are placed in institutional settings are usually those persons who do not have families. Most of these older persons had lost their families in the Great Patriotic War (World War II). As veterans of this war (for everyone was considered to have participated in this great patriotic effort), older persons are placed in the same category as war veterans or invalids.

With respect to nursing home care then, it is not surprising that a physician is at the head of the home; a dietitian is in charge of the kitchen; and a full dentist's office is located on the premises, dental care being regarded as part of medical care. The greatest problem lies in obtaining sufficient help in terms of aides. Every effort is made to place the work of the aides on a professional level, and to provide recreational activities such as membership in a chorus and attendance at lectures as a regular feature of the routine work. (This is also true for gerontologists. One afternoon at the Kiev Institute an exhibit and lecture on lithographs was held at the Institute in order to offset narrow professionalism.)

One facility located in Moscow consists of 10 floors and has a resident population of 910 persons, 20% of whom are between the ages of 80 and 100. Two of the floors are reserved for severely handicapped children and an additional two floors are reserved for the frail elderly. The resident population is made up predominantly of women.

The staff includes the director (a physician), 10 additional physicians, and 50 nurses. The number of aides fluctuates because of the labor shortage. The ratio is usually as follows:

1 doctor for every 100 patients

5 nurses for every 100 patients

1 aide for 8 bedfast patients

1 aide for 15 ambulatory patients

All of the medical needs of the residents are met on the premises. Dental, optical, auditory, and x-ray treatments are all available at the nursing home. Residents are sent to the hospital for surgical care.

A physical therapy laboratory is also a prominent feature, although also regarded as therapy is encouraging residents to care for their own rooms, to use their balconies for having tea and getting fresh air, to be active in the various work rooms, to take walks, and to participate in the national pastime of mushroom hunting. A forest adjoining the home is crisscrossed with paths and dotted with benches.

Psychological well-being is stressed through encouraging residents to bring personal possessions to the home, including items for religious devotion. Television sets and radios are in evidence, and the lace curtains and huge square pillows plumped up in the middle of the beds add to the homelike atmosphere.

The director indicated that there is little depression among the residents, and that they are encouraged to leave the home as often as possible for holidays and vacations in the many resorts and sanitoriums developed for the elderly by the state.

There is no attempt to set rules or regulations for the conduct of the residents, since the home is regarded as *indeed* their home. There is neither reality orientation nor scheduled games or activities. They do attend movies in town, dine in local restaurants, use their library, and attend the biweekly programs in the facility auditorium. Religious holidays are observed by the residents without criticism or censure.

The director made the comment, "You couldn't take Easter away from a Russian even if you tried."

Much emphasis is placed on preplacement counseling. During my tour of the home, the director called out to a woman seated among a group of women in one of the lounge areas, "Oh, Natalia Nikolaevna, remember how frightened you were, and how you insisted you would never come here to live?"

The women all nodded their heads.

Natalia Nikolaevna laughed, covering her mouth, "Oh, what a *fool* I was," she replied. "But I thought you would be like strangers!"

Everyone laughed, and we walked on.

At the end of the tour one of the residents was asked how she enjoyed living in the home. She turned and said with great feeling, "Kak v Hristoo za pazahi." (Like being tucked away in Christ's bosom.)

In some large metropolitan centers, those elderly, without family, who wish to live independently receive a variety of community services. There is the physician who makes house calls, and is aware of the elderly living in this region as part of his/her clientele. Free food, free linen service, and free housekeeping services, as well as free public transportation, are available.

Older persons with psychiatric problems are sent to special institutions and are not housed in the Dom Pistarelih (homes for the elderly). Such institutions are specifically designed to care for particular kinds of patients. For example, the Psychiatric Institute in Moscow treats only schizophrenic patients. Each institution has a profile, which means it treats and conducts research within limited parameters.

The section of the Psychiatric Institute in which the elderly female schizophrenics are housed is located within a large complex of buildings set in spacious grounds and surrounded by a high wrought iron fence. The wards look very much like back wards in American institutions: depressing, malodorous to the point of suffocation, understaffed, and with an overall air of hopelessness. The women were in large wards with beds lined up almost side by side. In some wards there were eight beds to a room; the sheets were worn and torn in some cases; the patients were dressed in faded old clothes; some were bedfast.

The activity room was stifling, with some 25 women led by an aide in making plastic flowers. There were 69 residents and a staff of 2 physicians and 4 nurses.

One woman said that she was being discharged the next day. Her comment was, "Thank God, they cured me. I thought I would never leave here when I arrived, but they really do their best to help you." The nurse in charge nodded her head in agreement, and added that most of the women in the wards would either be discharged or would be sent to other institutions according to their condition. The Psychiatric Institute is for short-term stays. The average stay is 3 months, though some of the women had been there a little over a year.

When there are also medical problems involved in the care of a patient, consulting physicians are available. Each patient receives a full physical checkup upon admission, including tests for hearing and vision. The physical and mental problems are treated concurrently.

When it is possible to keep an elderly psychiatric patient in the community, this is encouraged. Many such patients are treated at the outpatient clinics. However, when a patient misses one appointment, a home visit is immediately made.

One of the major health problems in the Soviet Union is overeating. This problem is especially prevalent in children, who of course grow up to be overeating adults. There is an overconsumption of sweets of every description. Not only is there a great consumption of sugar, but also of bread and fatty meat. Much of the food is fried, and breakfast often consists of sausages or kilbasi with thick slabs of butter on the bread.

Every official visit is preceded by a visit to the director's office for tea or coffee. The table is generally beautifully set with several boxes of chocolates, a huge plate of baked goods, a large bowl of the inevitable apples, a plate of cheese, a towering plate of bread, and tea. Endless, countless cups of tea. At the end of this refreshment break, the table will be barren. Every scrap of food will be eaten, even when only four or five have been at the table. They eat with energy and pleasure.

At every shopping area, and in some cities at every corner, there are huge confectionary stores for the sale of candy. In Kiev, where they are noted for a particular kind of cake or torte, it is not unusual to see people carrying three and four cakes in round boxes held together by string. When fancy boxes of candy are on sale at a hotel buffet, employee after employee will carry off as many as six boxes at a time.

Food habits, along with the chronic scarcity of some food items, were often brought up as serious gerontological concerns —as they sliced another piece of cake.

In the Soviet Union, excellence in geriatric medicine, like any other clinical discipline, is recognized as having to rest on a solid scientific foundation. It is regarded as essential that training programs in geriatric medicine include fundamental research in the problems of the aged, as well as in the processes of aging.

As a general observation, one could state that although both nations, the United States and the Soviet Union, face an increase in their aging population, the medical emphases in dealing with these problems differ considerably. In the Soviet Union, the priority in aging research is to find new knowledge with particular interest in ways of preventing, modifying, and even reversing some of the deleterious aspects of the aging process. There are constant references in the Soviet literature to "premature" aging. Such a search for new knowledge means fundamental understanding through research.

In the United States there is not such a national focus on research on aging, nor have the problems of aging been regarded in such a systematic fashion.

There are some commonalities, but a great number of differences in the kinds and types of problems older persons face in the United States and in the Soviet Union. These commonalities, as well as differences, can only be understood when viewed against the broader backdrop of cultural differences.

Part III

COMPONENTS OF HEALTH CARE

Just as medical care must be more broadly conceived, those components that contribute to the broad range of health care needs and services must also be redefined and expanded.

A realistic assessment of the status of health care of the elderly is a first step in determining what is currently being provided and the adequacy of such provision, as well as future need projections. The unit within which such care is commonly provided is the family, and the enhancing of the family's capacity to continue to provide such care is a task of major proportion that we must soon resolve.

Areas of particular concern, as they are vital to optimal functioning in terms of psychological and physical health, are exercise and nutrition. Negative stereotyping of older persons has restricted opportunities for physical education, and has thus markedly affected their health. Proper conception of the nutritional needs of older persons has not been developed, with the consequence that we are ignorant of the nutritional needs of persons as they grow old.

The requisites for normal healthy functioning in old age do not mean simply food, but scientifically determined dietary needs, and shelter does not mean solely minimal standards for existence, but the total environment, which incorporates persons within its concept.

Chapter 8

THE STATUS OF HEALTH CARE FOR THE ELDERLY*

Ethel Shanas

Some 30 years ago when I taught in the Committee of Human Development at the University of Chicago, we had a sequence in life span human development. The fall quarter was concerned with the child up to the age of two; winter quarter was devoted to later childhood and adolescence; spring quarter began with the young adult and covered middle age and old age too. Thus 30 years ago the child up to age two was important for study; the adolescent was important; but we paid little attention to the remainder of life following adolescence. Obviously, interest in life after adolescence is greater now than it was 30 years ago.

*The 1975 survey of the elderly was supported by the Administration on Aging, grant number 90-A-369, and the Social Security Administration, grant number 10-P-57823. The 1962 survey of the aged was supported by the National Institute of Mental Health and the Community Health Services Division of the Bureau of State Service, United States Public Health Service.

In discussing the status of health care for the elderly, a comparison will be made between people in this country in 1962, 3 years before health insurance for the aged (Medicare) was enacted into law, and in 1975, almost 10 years after the implementation of this legislation in 1966. The data comes from my nationwide studies of older people made in 1962 and 1975, and from a document prepared by Herman Brotman, special consultant to the Senate Special Committee on Aging, for the volume *Developments in Aging, 1977,*[4] a publication of that Committee. I shall begin with a definition of the elderly, then go on to discuss the Medicare legislation, the use of institutions by the elderly, the health status of the elderly as measured by functional assessments, and the current modes of care for the elderly sick. These topics are all important in understanding the status of health care for older people in the immediate future.

DEFINITION OF THE ELDERLY

Who are the elderly? In the United States we usually describe the elderly as those aged 65 years and over. This is really a designation selected by chance. We could have said that the elderly are those 55 and over; or we could have defined them as those 70 and over. But because our Social Security system pays total benefits to retired persons beginning at age 65, we have come to define the elderly as those aged 65 and over. There are now about 23 million people in this age group, and as Herman Brotman points out, they now total about one of every nine Americans. If we Americans all lined up, including babes in arms, one of every nine of us would be 65 and over.

As might be expected in a group this large, there is tremendous diversity among the elderly. Two thirds of them are under 75, one third are over 75. There are some two million Americans over 85 years of age. Because women outlive men, there are about 146 women for every 100 men among those aged 65 and over. The scarcity value of men increases with age so that among those over 85, there are about 217 women for every 100 men. As a result of this imbalance of the sexes, many programs in the service area such as senior centers and nursing homes become programs that serve primarily women.

Older Americans are a heterogeneous group. They include the poor and the rich, and they represent every ethnic group. They represent every shade of political opinion, and they also represent at least two generations of persons. We would not expect a 15 year old to be like a 40 year old. When we discuss older Americans or programs for the elderly, however, we are grouping together people of 65 and people of 90. These persons are not the same; the differences between these age groups are tremendous.

Such differences are easily illustrated by comparing two individuals born only 13 years apart. A person born in 1900 would be 78 years old in 1978, while a person born in 1913 would be 65. The individual with the 1900 birthday was an adult during the first World War and may even have served in the armed forces. The individual born in 1913 may remember the Liberty Bonds and the Armistice, but very little more about that great war. Even in the short span of time between 1900 and 1913, only 13 years, we find two people, both over 65, but whose social environments were completely different.

MEDICARE LEGISLATION

All most people know about health insurance for the aged, or medicare, is that someone files a claim for payment, and reimbursement for care is either allowed or disallowed. Last year I submitted to my insurer, Blue Cross, a form to cover the cost of my annual health examination, and I received $7.40. Since the cost of my annual health examination runs well over $100, I was puzzled. After a number of telephone calls to Blue Cross, I realized what had happened. They had punched in the wrong numbers, so they had my age as 71. As a result, almost everything on my claim came back saying, "Medicare will cover." Since I am not 71, Medicare covers none of my health cost.

But what will Medicare cover for those eligible? In 1965, the United States enacted into law a program of health insurance for the elderly, Title XVIII of the Social Security Act. This program, which went into effect in 1966, was designed to cover expenditures for the health care of persons 65 and over. Medicare has two parts. Under Part A, this legislation provides payments for hospital care; for posthospital extended care with certain restrictions; for care in skilled nursing facilities, again, with certain restrictions; and for certain home health visits, once again, with restrictions. Part B covers payment to physicians for services outside of hospitals and certain other out-of-hospital costs.

The bulk of long-term care for the elderly is not covered under this legislation, but under a companion program of medical assistance, Title XIX of the Social Security Act. The medical assistance act, Medicaid, functions through a cost-sharing program between the federal government and the 50 states. Medicaid is a means-tested Program and is available only to those described as medically indigent.

On July 1, 1975, the enrolled aged population in Part A of Medicare health insurance was about 22.5 million persons, or almost all the persons aged 65 and over. Those enrolled in Part B were about 97% of all eligible persons. The health insurance and medical assistance legislation together provide payments for long-term care of the elderly in both short-stay and long-stay institutions. Many persons expected that the enactment of Medicare and Medicaid would result in a great increase in the number and proportions of the elderly in long-term care institutions. This great increase, however, has not occurred.

Among the changes that have occurred since 1965 is that there has been a great rise in the cost of health care. According to *Developments in Aging, 1977,* between 1965 (when Medicare became operational) and 1976, the total health bill of the United States rose from $39 billion to almost $140 billion, a tripling of the cost of health care. This rise in cost is the result of a number of factors, of which Medicare is only a part. There have been vast technical changes in health care: the development of computer axial tomography (about $500,000 dollars per scanner); the use of sophisticated equipment to monitor heart patients; and so forth. The general level of inflation is also a factor: the salaries of workers in hospitals and nursing homes rose along with other salaries and wages; the costs of supplies and equipment in the health industry rose along with other costs. Between 1965 and 1976, there was also an increased use of health facilities not only by the aged, but also by many other segments of the population, especially the poor. Title XIX (Medicaid) does not cover only the elderly, but it applies to the poor of any age. With Title XIX, many people who needed health services and who were being denied such services, could now receive them.

In the period of which we are speaking, 1965–1978, the most rapid rise in costs was for hospital care. These costs rose from 34% to 40% of total health expenditures. Nursing home costs rose from 3% to 8% of the total, and other components increased accordingly. In 1975, the elderly, who constitute about 11% of the population, were responsible for almost 30% of all personal health care costs. This may be expected: it should be understandable that people who are frail and ill, not people in the prime of life, would be the people who have most need for health care.

According to the latest federal figures, only 68% of the health care costs of the elderly are paid through public programs. The remainder is paid by private insurers and old people themselves. The proportion of older people who are covered by private health insurance has risen since the passage of Medicare, and about 60% of all old people now have private health insurance that covers part of their hospital costs. In other words, having learned by experience what Medicare will actually pay for, old people now buy private health insurance to help cover their health care costs.

USE OF INSTITUTIONS

What happened to the use of long-term care institutions with the passage of Medicare? In the short run, there does not seem to have been a substantial increase in the proportion of persons aged 65 and over who live in long-term care facilities. The great majority of old people, about 95% live in the community: in their own homes, in the homes of their children, or with other relatives. They do *not* live in institutions, whether these be nursing homes, mental hospitals, jails, or institutions for the mentally retarded. In 1960, the census reported that about 4% of all older people were living in institutions. Medicare became operational in 1966, and in 1970 the proportion of old people living in institutions had risen to about 5%. The latest figures are that between 5% and 6% of the elderly are living in institutions.

The actual number of old persons residing in institutions, however, almost doubled between 1960 and the present. The number of able old people also increased, however, so that the proportion of old people in institutions did not show a great increase. My own estimates are that the proportion of old people who are likely to spend some time in a long-term care institution, including homes for the well aged, may indeed be as high as 1 in 10 of those alive during any 1 year.

From what limited studies are available, there is no indication that this 1 person in 10 (who may be living in some kind of group quarters, a nursing home or a home for the well aged) represents any greater use of such institutions by the elderly than was in effect before health insurance. In a nationwide study of the American public in 1957, 1 in ever 10 adult Americans reported that a parent, grandparent, or other close relative had spent some time in a home for the aged or a nursing home.

So far as can be determined, Medicare has not substantially increased the proportion of old people in institutions. Further, findings from nationwide studies indicate that Medicare has had neither an appreciable effect either in reducing the proportion of the elderly who are bedfast and housebound at home, nor on the overall health status of old people. In 1962, in a national survey, 8% of all old people were found to be bedfast and housebound at home in the community. That was about twice the proportion of old people in institutions. In 1975, about 10% of old people were found to be bedfast and housebound at home. Once again, this was about twice the proportion of old people in institutions.

HEALTH STATUS OF THE ELDERLY AS MEASURED BY FUNCTIONAL ASSESSMENTS

In both of these surveys, efforts were made to measure the functional capacity of old people. People were asked: Can you go out of doors? Can you walk up and down stairs? Can you get about the house? Can you wash and bathe yourself? Can you dress yourself? Can you put on your shoes? And, finally, can you cut your own toenails? In both 1962 and 1975, the same proportion of persons, two of every three, reported that they had no trouble with any of these items. Somewhat less than one of every three had some trouble, and a small group of people had a great deal of trouble: 8% in 1962, and about 6% in 1975. When dealing with 23 million people, however, 6% of the population is really still a large number of persons. They may be a small group compared to all the other elderly, but they are a large group for service providers.

Most old people are not sick. In 1975, of every 10 persons aged 65 and over, 5 said their health was good. About 3 said their health was fair, and 2 said their health was poor. Even among those 80 years of age living in the community, one half said their health was good.

Two things stand out at this point. First, despite Medicare, the sick and frail aged who are being taken care of at home substantially outnumber the sick and frail in institutions at any time, about two to one. Second, in the 9 years between 1966 and 1975, after Medicare was implemented, and in the 13 years between the 1962 and 1975 surveys, there was no major change in the functional capacity of older people.

CURRENT MODES OF CARE FOR THE ELDERLY SICK

What has changed since the early 1960s, and it is not solely due to Medicare, is the nature of physician practice as it relates to older people. Between 1962 and now, there has been a great rise in the hospitalization of the elderly. In 1962, the chance of an old person being hospitalized was about one in eight; now it is about one in six. The rate at which old people are being hospitalized has increased, but again, this is not solely due to Medicare. First, many more sophisticated medical techniques are available to the physician now, and in many instances these techniques cannot be employed on an outpatient basis. Perhaps some of them could be done on an outpatient basis if the patient is 25 years of age, but not for the patient 75 years of age. Second, this rise in hospitalization reflects a change in how doctors treat the elderly. Home visits to the elderly have all but vanished. The person who is sick at home now is told by the doctor to come to the office or to go to the hospital to be admitted.

The caretakers of people who are sick and frail at home—the bedfast and the housebound—have not changed. The people who need to have food brought into the house, to have meals prepared, to have their sheets changed, etc., are still being taken care of by their family members. Survey data indicate that overwhelmingly, in the case of a couple, the source of help with shopping, preparation of meals, and housework is a husband or wife. Couples help one another. Men take over traditionally female tasks as is necessary; despite the fact that those who are now the American aged were not raised in a period when both men and women were housekeepers and cooks. Husbands and wives of the elderly bedfast person, themselves elderly, are often unable to manage the total care of a spouse without outside help. Many report help from children who live outside the household; others report that they are assisted by a paid helper. These paid helpers might be from home help agencies; they might be from homemaker services; or they might be a person hired by the family to come in to bathe the sick person. There are instances reported where hospital nurses' aides engage in such part-time work. These persons serve as a kind of private consultant on problems related to the care of sick old people at home.

Adult children, whether in or outside of the household, are a major source of help in the care of the elderly. For widowed persons, adult children are often the only source of help.

About 25% of all persons in 1975 (excluding the bedfast) who said they had spent 1 day or more in bed because of illness in the year before they were interviewed, said that they had no one to help them. They somehow took care of themselves. Women are more likely than men to live alone; therefore, women are about three times more likely than men to say that they had no one to help them. There are increasing reports of people who say they are receiving help with meals, but the number receiving such services is very small compared to the number of people who are still in need of such services.

FUTURE CONSIDERATIONS

Health care for the elderly in this country is in a state of change. Programs for the future now being considered focus heavily on reducing the use of both hospitals and long-term care institutions. Where the public was once told that we should all see our doctor every year for annual physicals, we are now being told that unless we have a specific complaint we should not take up the doctor's time. The popular press reports speeches made by physicians saying that perhaps people should ignore minor symptoms and allow them to be treated by "tincture of time." All such advice is part of a program to reduce the use of hospitals by everyone, including older people.

There is also much discussion about reducing the use of long-term care institutions through the development of "alternatives" to institutionalization. It should be clearly understood that there are some among the elderly for whom the long-term care institutions is the best care solution. Instead of discussing "alternatives," we should be offering a broader range of health care options to older people. Such options should include day hospitals, adult day care programs, home health care, and homemaker services. There are many problems in the development of such programs. Some of these are funding problems; some of these are the kinds of problems that arise when people say, "We'll never get anybody to do that," or "We haven't got the staff."

Further, since the major caretakers of the elderly sick are their families, we in this country also need to consider programs and policies that will in some way make up to family members for the sacrifices they are making in providing needed services to older people.

REFERENCES

1. Gornick, M. Ten years of medicare: Impact on the covered population. *Social Security Bulletin, 39,* 3–21, 1976.

2. Shanas, E. New directions in health care for the elderly. In *Improving the quality of health care for the elderly.* Brookbank, J. W., (Ed.). Gainesville, Fla.: University Presses of Florida, 1978.

3. Shanas, E., Maddox, G. L. Aging health and the organization of health resources. In *Handbook of aging and the social sciences.* Binstock, R. H., & Shanas, E., (Eds.). New York: Van Nostrand Reinhold, pp. 592–618, 1976.

4. U.S. Senate Special Committee on Aging. *Developments in Aging, 1977.* Washington, D. C.: U. S. Government Printing Office, 1978.

Chapter 9

WORKING WITH THE FAMILY AND ENVIRONMENT*

Elaine M. Brody

Sorting out the dependencies that are due to advancing age—
that is, those that are intrinsic to the very processes of aging,
from those that are due to the psychological, social, and physical environment—is a task that has been a focus of research and
practice since the inception of interest in gerontology. Although
knowledge is far from complete, evidence to date indicates that
a significant proportion of the dependencies of older people is
not intrinsic but is environmentally induced. At the same time,
it cannot be denied that the general direction in old age is a
decline in the level of functioning. That is, there are physiologi-

*Some of the material in this chapter has appeared in two previous
published papers by Elaine M. Brody:

Brody, E. Environmental factors in dependency. In *Care of the elderly:
Meeting the challenge of dependency.* Exton-Smith, A. N., & Evans,
J. Grimley (Eds.). London: Academic Press; New York: Grune
& Stratton, 1977.

Brody, E. The aging of the family. *The Annals of the American Academy
of Political and Social Science, 438,* July 1978, pp. 13–27.

cal and disease-related changes that lead to some "normal" dependency. Even if scientific breakthroughs should eliminate the major diseases of old age, it is unlikely that the foreseeable future will witness cures of most of the normal dependencies. In other words, certain changes such as decline in visual acuity, in hearing, in muscle strength and so on, appear to be intrinsic to the very processes of aging.

If we recognize that for most people some decline is inevitable, then we have to re-examine the value judgment that is often implicit in attitudes toward aging; specifically, the notion that dependency per se is bad, while independence is good. Certainly, the number and the nature of supports that are required vary over one's lifetime, but normal healthy interdependence is a constant throughout the life span. For example, the young infant is totally dependent. As the young move through childhood and adolescence and gain more and more competence, they assume more and more responsibility for themselves. With maturity and parenthood, a care-giving role toward others is often assumed.

In the aging phase of life the individual again may experience some dependencies. However, at that point, the goals of care are very different from the goals of care in young children. The dependencies of old age are chronic, rather than transitional; they foreshadow continuing or increasing dependency. Chronicity dictates that the supports to maximize functioning must be sustained; they cannot be offered and then withdrawn. Our overall medical systems have not responded to the chronicity of the ailments of old age. Medicare, for example, was geared to a crisis-and-cure orientation. The number of home health visits was limited, as was the number of days in an extended care facility. Sustained need was not really taken into account.

Environmental influences are influential with all human beings, but older people are especially vulnerable. My colleague at the Philadelphia Geriatric Center, Powell Lawton, formulated what he calls the "environmental docility hypothesis."

What he said was, "As the competence of the individual decreases, the proportion of behavior attributable to environmental, as contrasted with personal characteristics, increases." We can draw an anology with respect to reliance on the social and psychological environment. Irving Rosow pointed out that the crucial people in the aging problem are not the old, but the younger age groups, because it is the rest of us who determine the status and condition of the old person in the social order.

In other words, attitudes towards aging and old people are the determinants on every level of what is done, or what is not done, to find solutions to the problems of older people. That new word that has been added to our vocabulary, "ageism," on the macro level determines such matters as priorities in the allocation of resources for income, for health and social services, for attention to housing and neighborhood environments, and so on. On the micro level attitudes creep insidiously into such incorrect psychodynamic formulations as "parent-child role reversal" and "second childhood." One is reminded of the injunction of Maggie Kuhn, the Gray Panther leader who says, "Don't turn old people into wrinkled babies."

If you listen to yourselves and to other people very carefully, you will realize that ageist expressions creep very subtly into our speech. There is a real need for consciousness raising about ageism, much like the process we are going through with respect to racism and sexism.

The vulnerabilities of children and their dependence on the social, physical, and psychological environment are expected. They are accepted and provided for by the family and by society. But in the main, the dependencies of old people have not yet been similarly legitimized.

Within certain parameters, children are programmed developmentally for a somewhat orderly progress in the reduction of dependence, and society distinguishes between normal, healthy dependence and that which is extreme or pathological. But the dependencies of older people appear with great variability and irregularity, over much wider time spans, and in different sequential patterns from those of children. In other words, there are really no normative patterns for evaluating dependencies in old age. Therefore, among the unsettled issues is determining exactly when and how, quantitatively and qualitatively, to provide the environmental supports that are necessary to avoid fostering unnecessary dependencies.

If we are to attempt to distinguish the "normal" dependencies from those that are environmentally induced we cannot assume that the slope of decline is so inevitable that we become therapeutically pessimistic. The goals really are twofold:

1. To identify and reduce what have been called the "excess disabilities" that are environmentally induced, and do not reflect the actual impairment. That is, actual function may not reflect potential function. The gap between actual and potential function may be an excess disability that has been environmentally induced. If we treat the excess disability successfully, the functioning level of the older person may rise.
2. To meet the residual dependency needs (those that are irreducible) in such a way as to maximize independence and functioning. The word *potential* is key, because with frail older people goals have to be somewhat different than they might be with younger people.

At this point, an apparent paradox should be mentioned: That is, meeting dependency needs, rather than fostering dependence, can foster independence. Misunderstanding of this concept has led to polarized attitudes about whether the aged should be urged towards independence, or whether we should make concerted efforts to meet their dependency needs. Some years ago Dr. Lawton divided all gerontologists into two groups. He said that one group consisted of the marine sergeant gerontologists. The marine sergeant gerontologists are the ones who say older people must be active and insist that they be independent. The other group of gerontologists, he said, were the bleeding heart gerontologists, who say, "Oh, those poor old frail people; let's give them lots of services."

The appropriate approach, of course, is somewhere in between. The balanced view now generally held is that appropriate services and physical environments, selectively provided, can maximize independence. The road to maximum independence is often paved with supports of various types. A very simple example would be an older person who is not ambulatory and is given a walker. If the walker enables that person to move around, it does not foster dependence. It fosters independence. Similarly, if you put an older person who is having difficulty managing in his own household into a housing facility that has appropriate services, those services are fostering independence rather than dependence.

I should like to touch upon problems related to the relocation of older people (i.e., the effects of environmental change) because they illustrate clearly and dramatically what the role of the environment can be. For the reader who is not familiar with the relocation effect, or transplantion shock as it is sometimes called, it is the negative impact on older people of moving them from one living situation to another.

Early in the 1960s a stream of research began that documented the negative effects of relocation, such as increased mortality and morbidity. This really startled gerontologists, and everybody began to get very worried about moving older people.

Other streams of research began subsequent to those early studies in which the moves studied were expanded from their original focus on institutionalized populations. Attention was then turned to identifying qualifying factors, such as the characteristics of the people who were most vulnerable to the relocation effect and the characteristics of the facilities from which they were moving or into which they moved. The reason for the move, its meaning for the mover, and the ways in which those moves were managed were also studied.

As data accumulated, it became apparent that the relocation effect could not be attributable to the simple fact that
somebody is moving from one place to another. It was found
that certain groups of older people were more vulnerable than
others. Older people who were physically ill, who suffered from
organic brain syndrome, who were depressed, or who were
moved involuntarily, were most vulnerable to the relocation
effect. In addition, disorganization during a move and immediately afterwards increased mortality. Many older people, in
seeking a solution to their problems, move several times in rapid
succession before they enter an institution. One can speculate
about the impact of such multiple moves.

Interestingly, other groups of researchers actually found
improvements in some groups of older movers, notably those
who were physically well and those who chose to move. For
example, in studying older people who moved into senior citizen housing, both Frances Carp and Powell Lawton found that
people who moved into such housing improved. They attributed the improvements to the facts that those older people
chose to move and did so voluntarily.

Other factors found to reduce or obviate the negative
effects of moving are the provision of opportunity for choice,
careful premove orientation to the receiving facility, counseling, and the participation of the older people in the decision-
making progress.

Considering the nature of our health system today, it is
easy to see what the dependency-fostering implications are of
a system in which the moves of many sick older people are
frenetic and chaotic. In hospitals, for example, a move may be
decided upon the day before the hospital is ready to discharge
the person, when the utilization review committee says, "Get
this person out quickly." Careful preparation may then consist
simply of calling a list of nursing homes to find an available bed.
The old person does not participate in the placement process;
there is no preparation and no choice. It is picking somebody
up like a lump of clay, and putting it down in another place.

We talk about the relocation shock in relation to older people. But if any of you have moved your households, and can think back to that time with the disorganization and the chaos and the sense of upset that you felt, it is easy to see that moving per se can be upsetting even when you are choosing to make the move and have something to say about it.

An even more interesting stream of research about the relocation effect concerns the effects of the environment itself. Morton Lieberman studied the effects of moving older people to institutionlike environments. He found that the negative effects did occur, and attributed them to the fact that the institutional environments to which they moved differed so radically from previous, more natural life-styles, that the older person's capacity to adapt was overloaded. When Lieberman reported on the relocation of some elderly mental patients, the strongest association with the outcome was the psychosocial milieu of the receiving environment. Patients placed in cold, dehumanized, dependency-fostering environments showed decline. In short, the characteristics of the environment itself influenced the outcome for the person moved.

Roberta Marlowe did a similar study in the San Francisco area, in which she assessed the environmental dimensions of two highly comparable groups of people who moved. She found that those two groups experienced diametrically opposed outcomes: One group did very well, and the other group "fell apart." She attributed that anomalous situation to the characteristics of the environments. Those people who improved went to environments that encouraged autonomy (that is, the residents' control over their own lives) and fostered privacy, personalization, and respect. Staff did not do things *for* the person that the person still had the capacity to do for himself. We all know that in many nursing homes, much is done for the patient that is theoretically in the best interests of the patient but is really in the best interests of the provider. It is often a lot easier to go down a row of rooms and dress people than to lay out clothes for one and permit the other to do what he possibly can.

That may save time, but it does not encourage the older person to do what he still can do for himself. Another of Marlowe's findings was that the environments to which the people who improved went encouraged social interaction and did not expect passivity; the residents were treated with warmth and positive attitudes. People who went to facilities with the opposite conditions withdrew and deteriorated.

The relocation literature documents the fact that lack of attention to psychosocial factors in care can be as lethal as a lack of attention to sheer medical care or to feeding people. Survival and subsistence do not constitute the whole answer when one is planning services.

Interest in the relocation effect has not been matched in gerontology with the same degree of concern for the opposite condition—that is, the negative impact of a failure to change the environment when a change is needed and wished for. We came across the negative effects of *not* moving, which clinicians have known about for many years, in doing a housing study at the Philadelphia Geriatric Center. We found that a group who continued to live under conditions of severe stress, declined very rapidly. For want of a better name, we characterized this phenomenon as the "immobilization effect": the negative effect of not moving when a move is needed. We conjecture that it can be produced by a lack of options, and in fact there are few living arrangement options available to older people. Alternately, it can be produced by psychological resistance to moving, even if there actually is an option. Some of the people we studied did not move even though they had both acute need and an option. Immobilization may also be caused by subtle declines that hamper the individual's capacity to mobilize the necessary psychic or physical energy, and lead to giving up.

Those observations fit with those of Morton Lieberman as a result of his study of older people on a waiting list for an institution. He found that the negative effects that are usually attributed to living in an institution actually occurred while those people were on that waiting list.

We feel that the immobilization effect can be caused not only by the older person's failure to move when indicated, but by the environment changing while the older person remains in place. Whether the change is in the individual or in the environment, the net effect is that there is not congruence between the environment and the older person's capacity to function within it. A major lesson that can be learned from the relocation literature is that the process by which the environmental change is effected and the nature of the environment are as important as the fact of change itself.

I would like now to turn attention to a very important part of the environment—the family. In the past there has been a basic error in the ways we looked at older people and their families, and the time is long overdue for it to be corrected. About 12 years ago there was a major conference on the family which was subsequently published as a book edited by Ethel Shanas and Gordon Streib. There seems to be a major resurgence of interest in the subject.

In my view, a major danger that we have to avoid is to look at the family as the provider of services to older people, rather than to view the whole family as the client. The needs of the total family must be evaluated if the older person is to be helped. An analogy can be drawn with the child guidance movement. When it was at its height it had a totally child-centered focus. When children were in treatment, the mother was regarded as the cause of all the children's problems; if only the mother behaved herself, then the child's problems would disappear. The child was the focus of treatment and the mother was engaged peripherally so that she would not sabotage the child's treatment. We now are in danger of becoming old person focused, just as then we were child-focused. In reality, the family is not simply a part of the older person's environment either to help the older person or to hamper planning. Rather, the family members themselves are just as directly affected, and their needs also require attention.

This approach is particularly important because of demographic changes, particularly the increase in the number and proportion of older people. The Bureau of the Census recently released data that document the increases in the population between 1970 and 1976. In those 6 years, the number of people 85 and over increased by almost 40%. Black people over the age of 85 increased by almost 62%! Historically, black people have not lived as long as white people. Thus very old black people recently increased at a more rapid rate than did very old white people; there is movement toward closing the gap between life expectancy for white people and for black people and other minorities.

The increase in the aging population is uneven, as the oldest part of the old population is increasing at a much more rapid rate than the total population of older people. People 75 and over, and 85 and over, are increasing much more rapidly than people between the ages of 65 and 74. What does this rapid increase among the very old mean?

If the very old are increasing most rapidly, and the projections indicate that the trend will continue, then the increases are occurring among those who are most vulnerable to the physical and mental assaults that result in the need for care and services. In the future, then, the people on whom the very old depend, their family members, will also be older. Even more often than today, the care-giving generation, which consists primarily of women in the next generation down (daughters and daughters-in-law), will be middle-aged, aging, and even old themselves. There are many, many families containing two generations of older people, the very old and the care-giving relatives. They are aging families.

The family life cycle has changed very significantly as a result of the increase in life expectancy. In contrast to all previous periods of history, modern couples have a relatively longer life time spent together, of which shorter segments are spent in childrearing. More old people commonly survive to grandparenthood. The data that have been collected in cross-national studies carried out by Ethel Shanas and her colleagues indicate that about four out of five of all older people have children and about 30% have great-grandchildren. The four-generation family is now a very common phenomenon. In the next century, zero population growth will have resulted in fewer older persons having living children, and of those, more will have only one child. In addition, rates of widowhood rise very steeply with advancing age. In the future, then, the increased number of very old people will have diminished resources for service provision from either spouse or from adult children.

There are, of course, many other implications for families. Family structure, for example, is usually described from the old down, so that we know how many adult children old people have, how many grandchildren, and how many great-grandchildren. There are relatively few data, however, on how many grandparents and great-grandparents people have. We do know, of course, that nowadays there are many, many more older people in the lives of young children.

The Social Security Administration did a study of family structure in the preretirement years, which gives us some information about the very elderly and their children. What it found was that at age 58 and 59 about 25% of the respondents had one or more surviving parents, although that dropped to about 12% at ages 62 and 63. Of people between the ages of 58 and 63, 10% had both parents living. Those data tell us something about the number of individuals in the age 58 to 63 group who have a surviving parent, but many of those individuals are married, and the spouse may also have a surviving parent or both parents, thus doubling the number of old people for whom a middle-aged or aging couple may have responsibility. Years ago Peter Townsend warned that the problem may shift from the problem of which of the children looks after a widowed parent, to the problems of how a middle-aged man and wife can reconcile dependent relations with both sets of children.

We are all familiar with the myth of family abandonment. That myth does not take into account this vastly different demographic picture, which means that families are responsible for a much larger number of older people. The myth calls to mind wistful older people who would love to be taken into their children's household, but who are rejected. That is really not so. The reality is that in the United States the preferred arrangement is to live apart from one's adult children. Most older people want to live near, but not with their children, a situation that has been described as a wish for "intimacy at a distance." They want constant contact, but they do not want to live in the same household. Choices about living arrangements for older people are really limited by two factors: health and income. When income and health permit, older people prefer to live apart from their families and do so.

We know who provides the care when needed by older people: it is the family. I need not belabor that point. The National Health Survey of Home Care again documented the fact that about 80% of the health services provided to older people are provided by adult children. In that study home care was defined as medically-related care such as bandage changing and injections, and personal care such as dressing, bathing, feeding, and cutting toenails. It is not known what those figures would have been if the definition had been broadened to include all of the other services that adult children provide, such as household maintenance, cooking, shopping, and transportation. Of course, there would be no way of calculating in percentages per population the emotional support, the response in crises, the interest and concern, and the knowledge that there is somebody to depend on.

There should be no misunderstanding. The fact that the family is, and always has been, the most effective provider of care in no way lessens the need for community services. The gross underdevelopment of such services in the United States is so well documented that it need not be elaborated here. They are needed to supplement the family services and to strengthen the family's capacity to do what it has always done willingly.

For each severely disabled older person in an institution, there are about two equally disabled in the community. It is quite clear that the older people in institutions do not have the social support network that their peers outside institutions have. Nationwide, only about 10% of people in institutions have a spouse. Those in institutions more often are divorced, widowed, separated, or had never married. Only about half of all persons in institutions have at least one adult child, in contrast to about four out of five old people in the community. And there are more old people in institutions who have only one child, in contrast to two or more children for those in the community. Old people in institutions more often are separated from children by geographic distance.

There have been several interesting studies carried out lately, one by the University of Pennsylvania and another by the General Accounting Office in the Cleveland area. What they found is that in contrast to people in institutions, people in the community who are severely disabled live in what is called a caring unit, with a spouse, or with adult children. The people in institutions who are equally disabled either do not have children, or the children may live at a geographic distance or be too old.

These data do not mean that all institutional admissions are appropriate. But grandiose estimates of the number of old people who could be discharged if only there were enough community services are simply not true. Whatever careful studies there have been on that subject estimate that about 12% to 18% of institutional admissions may be inappropriate. And those estimates are based on the assumption that the needed community services actually exist.

In our present system, the social support system too often is not taken into account in deciding what kinds of services people need. In some instances the assessment process is being grossly abused. New York, for example, recently instituted a point system for determination of eligibility for nursing home admission. An individual needs a certain number of points to gain admission. Points are assigned for such needs as those for help in toileting or in dressing, for impaired vision, and so on.

The individual's social support system is not evaluated. There is no assessment of whether or not there is family, how old the supportive family member is, whether the adult children are working, and the like. As a result, two old people with identical physical assessments may be assigned the same number of points: One may be a lone older person without any family, and the other may have a very rich network of support; yet they both get the same number of points. The system is being challenged in the courts, but in the meantime is creating chaos in the nursing home scene in New York.

We have lagged badly in this country in developing the needed community care services, although there has been some improvement. The health and social services are developing gradually, but still are grossly inadequate qualitatively and quantitatively. This contrasts, for example, with the Medicare system, which was virtually in place overnight. Despite Medicare's shortcomings, it is still a uniform system across the country. But health and social services have not developed that way. They are locally administered; they vary regionally, with multiple funding support at three levels of government, different eligibility requirements, and so on. The net result is a maze of services that may be duplicative and may vary greatly in quality and quantity from locality to locality. Complicating the scene is the focus on the individual rather than on the family at the point of service need. Resources to support the family, such as respite care and day care exist, but are by no means universally available.

Gerontologists are currently engaged in exploring the implications for society of demographic developments—particularly the emergence of at least two generations of older people. Bernice Neugarten characterizes the two generations of older people as the "young old," those from 55 to 74, and the "old old," those 75 and over. She points out that the young old are very different from the stereotypes of old age, and describes them as being "relatively free from traditional social responsibilities of work and family, relatively healthy, relatively well off, and politically active." For some of the young old, however, the aging of the family has added new stresses to their lives.

There is a major concern at this time about the impact of retirement and the productive or enjoyable use of time during the retirement years, which can sometimes be as long as 30 years. A lot of emphasis is placed on the need to develop new roles to replace the many central roles that have been lost by older people: roles such as that of worker, spouse, parent of growing children, and others. It is therefore ironic that a new role has been emerging for some of the younger generation of older people: that of caregiver to the very old. We really have to rethink the stages of life, because a new life stage has been added. The "empty nests" of some of the grandparent generations are being refilled with members of the great-grandparent generation, and the view of the retirement years as a time of rest and peace is for that subgroup of people unrealistic.

It is necessary that we proceed at an accelerated rate to develop community services that are inappropriately called alternatives. We have to sort out the kinds of services that the family will be able to continue giving and those that the community must provide. Another factor to be considered is the major social trend for more and more women to enter the job market and have commitments to careers. Some middle-aged women of this generation are being caught in a bind between the needs for care and services of their elderly parents and their responsibilities to their own children and to their jobs. As more and more young women have commitments to careers, when they reach middle age, they too will be confronted with such situations. Unless the community develops the services to help them, the stress will be severe and widespread. We are now carrying out a project at the Philadelphia Geriatric Center to try to develop information about what services need to be provided by the community to help these families.

I should also like to call attention to another group of older people. We must remember that not all older people have families. If there are about 80% of all older people who have at least one adult child, that means that there are 20% who do not have an adult child. And 20% of the current population of old people is about 4.6 million older people.

There are also older people who do have an adult child but not within a geographic distance close enough to allow them to provide day-to-day services. Thus about 7 or 8 million older people either have no adult child at all, or the adult child lives too far away to be of help.

Added to that group can be those older people who have had a history of poor relationships with family. As a family moves forward in time, relationships do not change radically. A young family that had poor relationships cannot be expected, when the parent is old, to suddenly mobilize itself to express close warm supportive relationships.

The plight of older persons without family is epitomized by the elderly man who came to my office about 20 years ago to apply for institutional care. I asked, "Why do you want to come into an institution? You look well. You tell me you are able to manage by yourself." He replied, "I am an orphan. My mother and father are dead."

While we must forge service links to families of older people, we must make special efforts as well to reach those who are without family and to develop the supports required by their unique needs.

Chapter 10

NUTRITION AND THE OLDER INDIVIDUAL

Donald M. Watkin

It is important that we realize the necessity of bringing together the diverse fields of nutrition, health, and aging. Every decade or so we get the impression that we are seeing the light at the end of the tunnel, but it only takes the next 5 years to make us all realize that that light is really not the end of the tunnel, but rather a freight train bearing down on us. With that in mind, this discussion will not result in solutions that you will be able to implement immediately. However, if you promote consistently the ideas to be presented for the next decade or two, you will have solutions to many problems now confronting those seeking to promote the concept of the nutrition/health/aging triad.

Nutrition's role in aging is misunderstood not only by consumers but by many health industry providers as well. This misunderstanding is created by an information vacuum among consumers and providers, into which have swarmed the faddists; the authors and publishers of the painless, effortless, quick, and not always safe diets that you read about so often; and the self-appointed consumer activists who exploit their political knowledge in scientific and medical realms in which they have had no education, no training, and very little experience. Those just mentioned compound an already difficult problem whose solution must come through the development of cadres of scientists, physicians, and allied health professionals who are knowledgeable and who can communicate effectively correct information to the public at large. I hope to persuade you to be realistic and to apply that realism daily when you teach others of all ages about the role of nutrition in the biology, sociology, economics, and politics of aging.

A distinction must first of all be made between those who are aging and those who are already old. Nutrition's roles are quite different in serving the needs and meeting the problems of these two groups. In government in particular, but throughout our society in general, the term aging is used improperly as a euphemism for the term aged. Hence, when the Administration on Aging administers a nutrition program, that program is specifically managed for the aged, and specifically excludes from its purview nutritional considerations of others who are aging, notably all others from conception onward who have yet to pass through the golden door at age 60.

Now if this situation comprised only the omission of needed research, education, and service among younger cohorts, it would be bad enough. However, this obvious deficiency is compounded by three additional faults which directly affect the Administration on Aging's Nutrition Program's ability to serve the aged themselves.

The first of these is the low priority given to those supportive services essential to a sound nutrition program for those who are already old: outreach, primary health care, and individualized education and counseling. The second is the promotion among the aged of those measures known to have proven value only when practiced throughout life, beginning when the individual is in utero. The third fault is the omission of research that is desperately needed to search the totally unexplored realm of the impact of nutritional intervention after age 60 on the health status of the elderly.

One comparison regarding this third fault is pertinent. The Administration on Aging, with resources of over $.75 billion dollars devotes nothing to research in nutrition, health, and aging, while the National Institutes of Health's National Institute on Aging (NIA) is supposed to cover all three fields with a total budget of $37.5 million. NIA in fiscal year 1978 devoted $1.4 million to nutrition research, and was overwhelmed by more than 400 new research proposals, potential support of which comprised only $500,000 of funds uncommitted during previous years.

Let us examine initially some problems faced by those working in both tiers of the fields of nutrition and aging: the tier serving those who are aging but not yet old, and that devoted to serving those already old.

Nutritional Needs of Those Not Yet Old

We are becoming a nation of older people, and that is all the more reason for paying attention to what those of us who are not yet old are going to be like in the year 2000 or 2030.

Almost a decade ago Dr. Alexander Leaf, Professor of Medicine at Harvard and Chief of Medicine at the Massachusetts General Hospital, Boston, asked me to have lunch with him to discuss the possibility of exploring scientifically the environmental factors contributing to the reputed longevity of persons living in a portion of Ecuador, in the Hunza District of West Pakistan, and in the Trans-Caucasian Republics of the Soviet Union. Since I was familiar with all these regions, and had had contact with knowledgeable scientists and physicians familiar with the longevity myths there, I gave Dr. Leaf little encouragement in regard to the value of such an expedition. Nonetheless, at the urging of a wealthy Boston physician and of the National Geographic Society, he devoted a good share of 1972 to seeking in these places the explanations for the reputed longevity. Early in 1973, his adventures were featured in the cover story of the *National Geographic* magazine. For 5 years thereafter, Dr. Leaf clung to the hope that the ages of those he had found in his "search for the world's oldest people" were genuine. However, in an issue of *Time* magazine his present disillusionment with his initial aspirations was then reported.

Unfortunately, one of our major problems is that the world is filled with persons still seeking the prize that eluded both Dr. Leaf and Ponce de Leon. When resources for the exploration of natural environments are lacking, man's ingenuity comes to the fore, as illustrated by the Nevada legislature's legalization of the production and distribution of Gerovital. (This is a procaine containing preparation developed by Dr. Ana Aslan, a Rumanian physician, sometimes referred to as the "Youth Drug" because of claims made that it is an anti-aging drug. Elderly people may benefit from it somewhat because it may act as an antidepressant, but all other miraculous effects have not been verified.)

The search for foodstuffs that influence aging is no less the subject of innumerable myths. Some are based on partial facts; others are derived from legend or manufactured from whole cloth. The saccharin controversy has generated much heat and much criticism of the FDA. However, virtually no attention has been paid to saccharin's role in the genesis of lifelong sweettooth problems for young children and adults, or to the high sodium content of foods and beverages that are dulcified with sodium saccharinate.

Government Programs

The extent of need among America's 32 million older persons does vary, but according to estimates by the Senate Select Committee on Nutrition and Human Needs, at least 8 million are in desperate need. The Nutrition Program authorized by Title VII of the Older Americans Act (NPOA) was conceived as a means of fulfilling the nutritional, health, educational, and social needs of the most needy 8 million. However, only a small portion of those in desperate need are being reached by even the meal service aspect of the program, and even more infinitesimal proportions by other elements of the Nutrition Program.

The concept on which NPOA is based was first recommended for implementation nationally at the 1969 White House Conference on Food, Nutrition and Health by that Conference's Panel on Aging. NPOA was conceived to use dining together as a center of gravity, drawing older persons to a central location where they could obtain not only a balanced meal but also primary health care, individualized education, and counseling on a variety of topics, as well as the popular and important opportunities for socialization and recreation with their peers. To date, federal efforts have been focused only on serving meals. Outreach, health science services, and education and counseling have received no emphasis at the federal level, and low priorities at most state levels.

With the Nutrition Program currently serving the average participant throughout the country only seven meals every 10 weeks, it is obvious that meal service alone is contributing little to the nutritional status of participants. It is also apparent that too few people in desperate need categories have been brought into the Nutrition Program through outreach.

For those already enrolled in the Nutrition Program, only the support of health, educational, and counseling services offer hope of providing information that will lead to higher levels of self-responsibility in promoting maintenance of or improvement of health and nutritional status. Personal self-responsibility is *the* key to resolution of the nation's health and nutrition problems for persons of all ages, beginning in early childhood.

Current knowledge if applied could resolve many of the problems we have been discussing, but presently such application is frequently blocked. Present-day economics demand, therefore, that each person be his/her own protector. Education as the first line of defense is a top priority in every health-oriented program.

It is essential that health industry providers distinguish clearly, in their own minds and in the formulation of applications to consumers, the two tiers of services: those applicable to the young aging and those applicable to those already old.

Effects of Change in Life-Style

Since 1966 we have seen a remarkable drop in the mortality from cardiovascular diseases. No one is quite sure why this has happened, but one of the few things that is known is that the life-styles of young people began to change about 1965. The best guess is that practicing good life-styles has contributed to this remarkable drop in the mortality from cardiovascular disease.

A statistical relationship has been demonstrated between dietary fat intake and the incidence of breast cancer. However, this can only be important to those people who are still young. There is no point in the light of present knowledge in telling someone who is 75 years old to cut down on dietary fat because it might produce breast cancer.

Life expectancy since 1900 has increased dramatically for the young, modestly for the middle-aged; but virtually not at all for both the young old and the old old. Here is revealed the real culprit so far as inducing mortality is concerned. The mortality rate doubles every 8 years after age 60. Hence, it can be said unequivocally that age per se is the greatest risk factor of all.

Dietary Effects

Many of these observations in humans have solid backing in the highly controlled studies performed in fish and rats by McCay and his colleagues at Cornell University half a century ago. They showed that lifelong restriction of dietary calories with maintenance of appropriate quantities of essential nutrients would increase the age at death. Now, although these observations are half a century old, no mechanism for the effectiveness of this calorie restriction has been established. The closest we have come to a possible mechanism are the proposals of Walford that caloric undernutrition heightens immune and diminishes autoimmune reactions when these parameters are displayed as functions of age.

NUTRITIONAL NEEDS OF THE AGED

Having reviewed the needs of those aging but not yet old, let us now look at the needs of those who have already passed through that golden door at age 60. Health tops the list, followed by education and income maintenance. Nutrition is not considered separately here because it is a major component of health and of education, and its provision in appropriate quantity and quality is dependent upon resolution of other problems.

Skyrocketing Health Costs

The personal and societal costs of health problems among the nation's aged have risen dramatically. Costs tripled between 1966 and 1974 and took off in an almost exponential rise in the next 4 years. Totaling about $1,200 per year in 1974, the costs for the elderly were greatest when compared with other age cohorts regardless of the category of care provided.

In terms of specific nutritional needs, calorie intake should be reduced, but the levels of protein, vitamins, minerals, and trace elements should remain constant. This means that an older person requires a diet of high nutrient density. Diets high in nutrient density and the foods they contain are costly. Hence, the planning and preparation of low-cost diets that provide adequate nutrition require the maximum skill of professional nutritionists.

Now that some of the problems in lifetime perspective have been reviewed, let us look at potential solutions.

Need for Nutritional Education

Popular conceptions are one thing, but the reality rub-in is another. Nutrition, health, and gerontology or aging are agglomerates, each involving a multitude of disciplines: clinical, biologic, economic, social, political, etc. Rather than thinking of them as discrete entities, it is more appropriate to think of them in exponential terms. When an application brings together these three disciplines, the result has a magnitude of complexity equivalent to the sum of the exponents of the component parts, if not their product.

The challenge in any application, and here the NPOA is used as an example, is to assemble the agglomerates with already huge dimensions into an integrated whole whose complexity far exceeds that of its component parts. The need to disseminate knowledge through education and to provide the means by which this knowledge may be effectively applied represents an immediate challenge. The knowledge is available, but it is not always well distributed among health industry providers, let alone among consumers. Its application to date has been grossly deficient.

Ways must be found to bring nutrition, health, and aging together in an integrated triad. No one component of this triad should stand, or can stand, alone.

Early in 1977, publication of *Dietary Goals for the United States* by the Senate Select Committee on Nutrition and Human Needs was a/ happening of great significance to nutrition and aging when viewed in lifetime perspective. The promulgation of these goals produced a storm of protest from professional societies and individual nutrition scientists who viewed as very premature public health pronouncements based largely on concepts of disease control. However, the controversy has probably been the best thing for nutrition in over a decade.

Scientists, physicians, allied health professionals, politicians, media persons, and members of the public have had their say. Interest in nutrition and its relation to health is high. The Senate Committee has indicated its own willingness to alter the goals as new information becomes available. All told, the controversy has made all Americans more nutrition and more health conscious, and therefore, the educational value of the promulgation of these goals has been enormous.

As one example, the publication of the sodium content of processed versus fresh foods has revealed much to the American public. Fresh peas have practically no sodium in them, but after they are canned, they contain 10 milliequivalents of sodium in each 100-g edible portion. The sodium content in many drugs has been a matter of concern. The *Wall Street Journal* recently printed a front page announcement that the Commissioner of the FDA was about to implement a requirement that labels quantifying the sodium content of both foods and drugs be applied to all food and drug products. This is a development of importance to all the people who are already old and on salt-restricted diets, as well as to others in younger age groups who seek to limit dietary sodium as a measure designed to prevent hypertension.

Nutrition as Therapy

Among those already old, nutrition may play, in spite of some of the things already discussed, a truly life-saving role, especially when the older person is afflicted by an acute illness or accident. Such events are associated with decrease in appetite, increase in stress, and even by sensations of nausea and occasionally vomiting. These symptoms lead many elderly persons to reject food and fluid. Such rejections in turn lead to dehydration, extracellular and intracellular electrolyte disturbances, and, in relatively few hours, depletion of the already diminished protein reserves of older persons.

Hence, among the aged, prompt treatment of the underlying pathology must be accompanied by equally prompt provision of fluid and of nutrients. This can be accomplished by small frequent (hourly or half-hourly, if necessary) servings of nutrients and water. These feedings need not comprise bullion, juices, gelatins, etc., but rather should be composed of what may be called regular food properly seasoned to augment its acceptability. If such food is unavailable or impractical, any combination of appropriate nutrients will perform the essential task.

Aged persons do respond to nutrient administration. Prompt therapy for the primary disease or trauma must be accompanied by equally prompt fulfillment of nutrient and water needs in acute illness and accident, if excessive morbidity and mortality (not to mention cost) are to be avoided.

THE NEED FOR RESEARCH

This discussion to this point has dealt primarily with the more effective application of what knowledge is already available. Obviously, there is a veritable universe of information still to be acquired in the realm of nutrition and aging; this demands exploration and application to human development from before conception to the time of death.

Among those already old, two examples will illustrate the type of biochemical studies indicated. Much more investigation is needed in calcium homeostasis with particular reference to its role in the osteopenia of old age in the disease of osteoporosis. Recent collaboration by representatives of the University of Wisconsin (Madison), the Mayo Clinic (Rochester, Minn.), and Creighton University (Omaha, Neb.) has suggested that agewise decrements in renal function correlate with comparable decrements in the transformation of liver-produced 25-OH vitamin D_3 to 1,25 $(OH)_2$ vitamin D_3 in the kidneys. This recent important lead has already led to clinical investigations using 1,25 $(OH)_2$ vitamin D_3 analogues in the management of osteopenia from whatever etiology.

In studies from New Zealand, a land which has a low selenium content in its soil already, the elderly have been found to have lower whole-blood erythrocyte and plasma concentrations of selenium than young control subjects. In addition, the lower selenium concentrations correlate well with lower erythrocyte and hemoglobin concentrations of glutathione peroxidase, an enzyme vital to the effective function of all cell membranes throughout the body. This certainly is a topic that deserves much further investigation, since we know that one of the major causes of cell death is malfunction of cell membranes, and since cell death is the major phenomenon characterizing biologic aging.

But what about more basic research? Alex Comfort has proposed an ultimate human survival curve, which presumes a technical lifespan of about a century, no different from that of all recorded history. Walford, on the other hand, envisions a technical lifespan of 140 years to be achieved by more research and through more application of that research. Walford envisions a change not only in technical lifespan—that is, the oldest age to which a member of the human species is known to have lived—but also other changes resulting from treatments beginning very early in life. Puberty, for example, would be postponed until the 20s; menopause, until the 70s. Diseases of old age would be delayed, and exposure to them would cover fewer years than now. Walford, an immunologist, looks to recent advances in immunologic research to be in the vanguard of this drive toward a new technical lifespan and a new spectrum of development from before conception until death.

What about less esoteric research that might lead to an older average age of death, assuming the technical lifespan of about 113 years, which is what it is now, remains unaltered? Life-style adjustments, particularly in regard to lifelong nutrition practices, are of proven effectiveness. Of the seven life-style changes of practices recommended by Belloc and Breslow, five of them have direct bearing on nutrition. We have already seen what has happened, presumably from changes in life-style that have resulted in the past 10 to 12 years in the terms of the death rate from cardiovascular disease. The Framingham and Hawaii data regarding high-density lipoproteins suggest the mechanism through which life-style changes, which diminish gluttony and increase physicial activity, may work even among those who are already old. In addition, many lives of those already old can be saved from premature death by prompt treatment including, especially, attention to nutrition and hydration.

THE NEED FOR ATTITUDINAL CHANGE

Attitudes can be changed. More realism, more humanity, and more knowledge of the capabilities of the elderly by health providers can help eliminate counterproductive attitudes among those already old. The attitude of the late Supreme Court Justice Holmes suggests a very rational approach: "Some people as they approach 70 begin to read the Bible and prepare to die; others prepare to live until they are 90. Now if the ones who prepare to live to 90 die at 70, they won't know the difference, but if the ones who prepare to die at 70 live until they're 90, the last 20 years will be hell." Holmes, by the way, is notorious in Washington for his frequently repeated expression as a nonogenarian to his law clerks when he saw an attractive young lady. It went something like, "Oh, to be 70 again."

About the most counterproductive attitudinal pathology is that characterized by too much pride to take advantage of resources made available by society to relieve the burdens of old age. Many older persons refuse such help as is available through Medicare, Medicaid, the Nutrition Program for Older Americans, public assistance, and the Supplemental Security Income Program, and many even say they will not tap the social security fund to which they have contributed all their working lives. Fortunately, a recent law signed by the president increases the retirement age and abolishes retirement age for federal employees. This will be a real test of the proficiency and the

productivity of the elderly. Now that a major block to employment in old age has been removed, it will be very exciting to
observe the statistics and the changes in those statistics that will
occur over the next decade.

But what about those in younger age cohorts and particularly the youth of the nation? These cohorts must be inspired
by the example of those already old that old age can be a
productive time, a worthwhile time, and a time that is lots of
fun. Practicing appropriate life-styles and obtaining appropriate health care, as indicated, can assure the highest probability
of effective longevity.

IMPROVING CURRENT PROGRAMS

Finally, what can be done to get more effectiveness, including cost effectiveness, out of our present national Nutrition
Program for Older Americans? We now have over 10,000 sites
and a budget including all resources of almost $500 million; yet
there are many problems.

First of all, some form of objective evaluation is absolutely
essential. This need was illustrated by a recent experience in
which 6,000 older people distributed among 20 Nutrition Program projects in 17 states participated in an exploration of the
acceptability of a limited use supplemental food (LUSF). This
is basically skim milk powder with vitamins, trace elements,
and corn syrup solids added. The 6,000 were asked only for a
report on acceptability; that is, do you like it or not? However,
most reported additional long lists of amazing results. Not only
did LUSF improve the hair, strengthen the nails, and make the
cheeks pinker; it also improved the sex life, increased energy in
the morning, and promoted more restful sleep at night!

Obviously, to evaluate the effectiveness of any of our
health-oriented programs, we must have more objective data.
We cannot rely on subjective reports from older persons. Also,
a much higher priority than is currently practiced must be given

in the Nutrition Program to primary health care at the Program sites; to education and counseling, individualized to meet the needs of each person; and to more effective outreach, to bring in the people who are really in need and minimize the number of affable, gregarious, affluent, well-transported, and church-going people who now comprise the majority of participants.

Finally, some mechanism must be established to enable the older people participating in this program to have far more contact with the young. During such contacts, the elderly can demonstrate to the young that old age is really an enjoyable and productive time of life. They can also point out mistakes they have made that the young people might be able to avoid to make their longevity more effective.

Let me summarize by saying that methods now being used to bring together the diverse fields of nutrition, health, and aging are too Balkanized to be effective. The nutrition/health/aging triad concept needs to be adopted universally, particularly for the aged; health care and nutrition services must be combined. Younger aged cohorts need far more information translated into applied knowledge about health, nutrition, and aging. In addition, they need to develop by observing good examples a far better image of old age. Finally, far more research is needed. Research is, for all ages, the most valuable service that can be provided. This should be reflected in the budgets of governments at the federal, state, and intrastate levels and in the budgets of all nongovernment agencies and the other organizations devoting their attention to the complex fields of nutrition, health, and aging from before conception to death.

In conclusion, let me emphasize a concept of vital importance to those who are already old. The nutritional needs of the elderly do not stand alone. They are intertwined with other factors and attitudes affecting health. Nutrition must be considered only as part of a constellation of circumstances affecting the health of the elderly.

Chapter II

PHYSIOLOGY OF EXERCISE AND AGING

Herbert A. deVries

I should like to discuss some new health concepts, particularly in relation to the changing nature of disease; and as so often happens, there is good news and there is bad news.

The good news is that our friends in the medical profession have done such a superb job over the last 50 years that they have virtually eradicated most of the infectious disease processes, such as influenza, pneumonia, bronchitis, and tuberculosis. The bad news is that as these infectious diseases have receded into the dim past, we are now coming to grips with a new group of diseases loosely termed the degenerative diseases: heart disease, cancer, arthritic problems, etc.

Looking at the very important question of health costs, I will present the bad news first. In 1965 our national bill for health and health care, etc., was $39 billion; in 1975, it was $118 billion. That is a threefold increase in just 10 years' time.

The good news is that our daily habits—our life-style, if you please—appears to be much more important to our good health than anything that anyone else could do for us.

I should like to cite, in some detail, the work done by our colleagues at UCLA, particularly Dr. Breslow and his colleague, Dr. Belloc. They set up a study with the California Department of Health at the human population lab in Alameda County, in which they studied the effects of individual health practices on health and mortality. This is the first time we have collected any data that specifically deals with morbidity and mortality with respect to health practices. The following items were taken into consideration:

Do you usually sleep 7 or 8 hours?

Do you usually eat breakfast regularly?

Do you eat between meals?

Do you maintain normal body weight?

Do you engage in regular vigorous exercise?

Do you use alcohol?

Do you smoke?

Their findings, in my mind, were extremely important. They found the highest mortality rates were for the groups that (1) were 10% or more underweight; (2) were 20% or more overweight; (3) were cigarette smokers (one of the important factors in increasing mortality rate). Equally important were lack of physical activity and irregular meals. Interestingly enough, with respect to sleep, they found a dichotomy of effects between the male and the female. The mortality rate was higher for the women who slept more than 9 hours; for the men it was higher for those who slept less than 6 hours. Of course, the mortality rate increased with the heavy use of alcohol, although their data corroborated the classic data with respect to alcohol, and that is that the person who is worst off is the heavy drinker. The teetotaler does not do as well as does the individual who drinks in moderation (defined as about one drink per day).

The more health practices observed, the lower the mortality. There were nine times as many men who died over the

5-year period among those who could answer appropriately on that UCLA study questionnaire to only three or so questions, compared to those who could answer appropriately to six or seven of the seven. The women didn't demonstrate quite such an advantage, probably because women are better off than men to begin with due to their greater life expectancy. Their advantage, however, is still 3.6-fold.

Looking at life expectancy, the males who could answer appropriately to six or seven of the questions had 11 years better life expectancy at age 45. The women had 7 years better expectancy. At age 65, which is of greater interest to many of us, both men and women had a better life expectancy of 7 years if they could answer yes to six or seven of those questions. Also noted was a positive relationship between physical and mental health regardless of sex, age, or even income. The same thing held true for social health.

The important conclusion to be drawn here, in my mind, is that to a very great extent we now control our own health destiny. What we do to and for ourselves is far more important than anything anyone else could do to or for us. Let us look more specifically at good health practices.

We feel in our work that the three major areas contributing to what we call positive good health, both in youth and old age, and all through the ages, are these:

1. Maintenance of good physical fitness; physical conditioning brings about all kinds of improvements that have been well documented, so far as cardiovascular and respiratory functions are concerned.
2. We are very concerned about nutrition, with respect to the maintenance of appropriate body weight.
3. Another area of concern for us is relaxation.

I will limit my discussion to these areas of exercise physiology and devote some attention to relaxation and some of the experiments we have conducted in that area with older people.

First, with respect to the use of exercise for the elderly, we became interested around a decade ago in the very basic question of just how trainable is the older organism. It had been said by a physiologist for whom I have great respect that in all probability, if an individual had not conditioned himself in youth, then beyond the age of 40 or 45 there is no likelihood of bringing about any improvement. Well-trained physiologists were drawing these conclusions, but they were still at the opinion level.

That did not correspond with what we had seen regarding adult conditioning, and there were good data already in the literature showing that the level of trainability of the middle-aged is still virtually as good as in youth. We set about looking at this question with respect to the elderly and trying to learn what we could about the important "how-to" questions. We immediately found that there was a problem of getting large numbers of older subjects into our laboratory at the University of Southern California. Many organizations were very happy to send volunteers, but the first question was always, "When would you come to get them?" Since I really didn't have any notion of getting into the transportation business, we took the mountain to Mohammed. We built a mobile laboratory and took it down to Laguna Hills, where we had access to 14,000 people whose average age is about 70 years. With a little solicitation and a little urging and coercion, we finally found some 112 willing older volunteers. We then went to work on them, after having given them a medical examination and a rather comprehensive set of physiological tests.

We were very interested in blood pressure, of course, because earlier data on middle-aged men had shown that this was one of the parameters that did respond in the proper direction. And we were also interested in body composition, and since in this age bracket over 50% of the people do not swim, the usual laboratory procedure of underwater weighing is somewhat traumatic. Also, it takes a lot of time. So we used the simpler skin-fold technique to get an estimate of the body composition in terms of percentage of fat. We also measured relaxation by electromyographic techniques. It had been hypothesized by many people that exercise is an excellent way to achieve relaxation.

Then we put them on the simple bicycle ergometer and got some quick and dirty data, as we call it, on just what approximate kinds of fitness levels we had, and we did that by simply relating work load to heart rate.

Once having that kind of data, we then went into the more complete examination, which involves pretty much what the cardiologists call a stress test, in that we were taking the electrocardiogram at every increasing work load; we were also doing gas analysis and getting measurements of oxygen consumption, carbon dioxide output, ventilation, etc.

We also measured cardiac output—the amount of blood put out by the heart each minute—by indirect techniques. With these measurements in our possession, and knowing a little bit about these people, we then took them out to the field; and in groups of approximately 20 to 25 we started an exercise program for them.

The exercise program was designed to accomplish mainly cardiovascular conditioning. It was built around endurance-type exercise, but to keep it from being deadly boring, we also used calisthenics to challenge them a little bit. We also gave them a little practice at balancing. Balance functions are among those that we lose predictably with age, and the exercises were meant to build strength and flexibility. We also had some aquatics. Our goal was to take a quick look at just how much possibility there was for bringing about hypertrophy and strength gains in older men.

Push-ups were modified so that even the poorly conditioned elderly people could do them. By allowing bending of the knees, we can cut down on the amount of load on the arms and make it a lot easier.

We also used some exercises from yoga. We call them static stretching, however, because we have generalized upon the neurological principles of yoga and then implemented them in many other ways with the main purpose of preventing and eliminating muscle problems in older people. It works with the young as well. The basic idea is that much of the soreness that we experience 24 to 48 hours after exercise is the result of minor muscle spasms; this we have found from electromyographic research. This is fairly easy to prevent, by simply making certain that the individual never leaves the workout area without having stretched completely all the muscles that may have been involved in the exercises. We saw very little incidence (maybe one or two out of the class) of any kind of muscle problems at all. But we leaned over backwards in trying to prevent it.

We also expanded the program to the use of the swimming pool. Some of the subjects developed problems with their feet, knees, or ankles over the years, and might not have been able to continue the jogging on which we based our program. Consequently, we wanted to teach them to swim well enough so that they could use the swimming pool as a conditioning medium, even if they had some orthopedic problems. They enjoyed this; not only that, but we were amazed that with these older gentlemen, none of whom were competent swimmers when we started (some of whom were virtually beginners), we found no need to modify our methods of teaching swimming and could employ the same methods we used with college-age people. I have no data to show that learning curves were just as good as those of college-age students, but I can say that there was no obvious difference.

The jog-walk is the meat and potatoes of the exercise program. We started with a very moderate dose in which each man jogged 50 steps, then walked 50 steps; we did this 5 times. That was the program for the first day, along with the calisthenics, etc. The second day he did it 6 times; the third day, 7. When he got up to 10 times, we then cut down the walk interval by 10 steps and started at 5 again. They then started at 5 sets of 50 jogging, 40 walking. This turned out to be a fairly practical approach to the problem; we found that, with a few exceptions, the men could live with this regimen. Within 6 months to a year, we had most of them going a mile without stopping. That is a pretty good bit of jogging for previously sedentary men in their 70s and 80s.

Now as to the results: The controls whom we tested before and after a 42-week exercise period were compared with the experimentals who stayed with the exercise program. The single most important parameter was the measure of oxygen consumption per unit heartbeat, which is a fairly good reflection not only of metabolic processes, but also of stroke volume and heart dimensions in particular and heart function in general. This parameter improved in the experimentals by 29%, a very large improvement. We do not expect any more than that with the young.

The data on vital capacity—i.e., the greatest amount of air you can exhale after a maximum inspiration—also improved very significantly, by approximately 19% to 20%. The largest percentage improvement, also very significant, was in the ventilation at maximum exercise, which improved by 35%. This was a very big improvement indeed. Thus we are saying that the average experimental after 42 weeks of conditioning was able to ventilate 35% more liters per minute than when he started. Of course, the controls did not change.

Percentage body fat we have to regard as an estimate only, since we used skin folds instead of underwater weighing. It showed the changes we expected, however. We found a significant decrease in percentage fat, and there was no dietary modification. In fact, we did our level best to convince the members of the program not to modify their diet, because we wanted to relate cause and effect with respect to the exercise program, unconfounded by other changes.

Our older men after conditioning 42 weeks were about as good in aerobic capacity as the average unconditioned young man of age 40 or so. I am not saying that we took 70 year olds and made 40 year olds of them. What I am saying is that it is possible to compensate for at least some of the losses by age through physical conditioning. That is not to say that we have reversed any of the basic age changes, but at least function is improved. Thus I think it bears emphasis that the potential for improvement in the older people, stated on a relative basis, is just as good as it is in the young.

After having collected these data on the men, we repeated the same sort of study with a somewhat smaller sample of the women from the same population. Essentially the data were very similar, with one important distinction. Women did not show any improvement in respiratory functions, whereas that had been the largest single improvement in the men. I have no data to elucidate that; all we can surmise at the present time is that women do not grow stiff at the same rate as men do. It is logical to believe, though there is not much evidence, that the thoracic wall compliance (the elasticity of the chest wall) has not suffered as much in the women as it has in the men. Consequently, there wasn't as much room for improvement. Such an explanation, however, is only a guess at best.

We have been a little technical up to this point. But there is a simple formula for gradually working up to good physical fitness with respect to aerobic capacity. We learned over the years with the collaboration of many others and the corroboration of other groups, that, surprisingly, walking is an excellent exercise. Jogging is not even necessary if the individual is not highly conditioned to begin with. With a typical sedentary group, brisk walking provides a very good stimulus. This is just a very simple progression that we have used successfully; there are many other ways to go about it. But if you can bring an older group to the point of walking a minimum of 30 minutes, five or six times a week, you will be accomplishing a great deal in the way of aerobic conditioning.

We also took a hard look at the matter of joint mobility. One of my graduate students, Dr. Betty Chapman, for her doctoral dissertation used electronic instrumentation to measure the torque required to passively oscillate finger joints. I should like to emphasize that we like to stay clear of subjective reports. What we like to have is the hard data from instrumentation, which provide us with objective figures. The first finding was obvious: The older individuals did, in fact, have much stiffer finger joints. The second part of Chapman's procedure was to exercise the hands, using essentially the principles of progressive weight training through the use of the devices by which subjects move the fingers in lifting some weights. She found very significant improvement both in the old and in the young with respect to joint stiffness. This is just one set of joints, but I have no reason to think that it should not be generalized.

If the older group is already in fair physical fitness, then the walking will not provide sufficient stimulus. Then we have to get into the jog, or jog–walk program.

To use the jog–walk program or head toward a jogging program for older people, it is important to include a medical examination. It is of great help to have some physiological monitoring going on as well, even if it is only simple bicycle ergometer tests relating heart rate to workload.

With respect to the prescription of exercise or the design of exercise programs for older people, one of the early questions we needed to consider was, what type of exercise, before we could even think about intensity. Is there a difference if we use isometric contraction, static contraction, dynamic contraction? We got the gross picture between the extremes very quickly: Isometric exercises drive blood pressure up very rapidly. We then made a somewhat finer comparison in which we started looking at three different kinds of exercise, involving (1) varying amounts of large muscle activity; (2) small muscle activity; and (3) dynamic and static contractions. We used walking on a treadmill or treadmill-type walking; cycling on the bicycle ergometer; and crawling on a machine that had been programmed for crawling for other purposes. In any event, the walking represented the rhythmic use of large muscle groups and virtually no static or isometric contractions. The bicycle ergometer (or cycling in general), on the other hand, also used rhythmic activity of large muscles, but you may be surprised to know that there is a considerable component of isometric contractions through the arms and shoulders. Finally, the crawling had a very heavy commitment on the part of small muscles of the forearms, the upper arms, and the shoulders.

What we wanted to do was maximize the general amount of exercise that the whole body is getting with a minimum amount of stress on the heart. This is because with the older population we never know how much function has been lost. The best exercise, from that standpoint, is the very natural, normal exercise of walking. And the same thing holds true pretty much for running. The point is to stay with exercises that are rhythmic in which one does not hold a contraction for a long period of time. The best exercises are those in which we use large muscles; those to be avoided are the ones in which we use high percentages of the capacity of small muscles. We want to avoid the exercises that involve static contractions.

We wanted to get some information about the threshold: How hard do we really have to work the older individual to start bringing about an effect on his aerobic capacity? What we found was that a little over 40% of our capacity is sufficient to start bringing about a training effect in sedentary older people. This is very important, because 40% for the elderly can be achieved without jogging; it can be done by walking. Thus the relatively sedentary and unconditioned can walk themselves up to the threshold value and above, bringing about a conditioning effect.

This is the method we use in prescribing exercise and in monitoring the stressfulness of various kinds of physical activities. Percent of heart rate range is arrived at by subtracting the resting heart rate from the exercise heart rate and dividing that by the total range, which is the maximum heart rate minus the resting heart rate; we then multiply by 100 to get percent.

Thus we can arrive at a fairly good reflection of the percent of the individual's capacity at which he's working. This has many advantages over most other systems in that it provides a very good input as to how the activity is affecting the individual under the conditions that exist on that particular day; such input is not provided by systems such as the aerobic point system.

Here is our method of setting up an exercise program. We take a hypothetical individual of 73 years of age with a resting heart rate of 70 beats/minute. First we need to know his maximum heart rate. Knowing very little about the man, we do not take him to a maximum exercise heart rate; rather, we estimate it from his age, using the simple rule of thumb that maximum heart rate is approximated by 220, minus the age. So for the 73-year-old individual, 220–73 gives us a maximum heart rate of 147; and the range is between 147 and 70, or 77 beats/minute. We then take 40% of that value and add it to the resting value; and we come up with the heart rate that is minimum for him to attain any measure of physical condition. In this case that value carries out to 101 beats/minute. That value is roughly what you would get from moderate walking under normal ambient conditions.

Then we give him a target heart rate at which we believe the best possible results are attainable, and we use 60% of the range for that; thus, using the same procedure, we arrive at about 116 beats/minute. We achieve this value with brisk walking in men and women of this age bracket over a period of 20 or 30 minutes. For the maximum we would use 75%, leaving a nice big cushion between that heart rate and their actual maximum. Going to maximum is counterproductive in the older organism.

I should like to touch on the matter of relaxation. The importance of this area is perhaps best brought home quickly by pointing out that in the United States we spend over a billion dollars a year on tranquilizing drugs. The use of drugs to alter attitudes and emotions has become very popular. But there is no tranquilizing drug, or any other drug used for that purpose, that is free from undesirable side effects. The narcotics, such as morphine, are addictive. The sedatives, such as phenobarbital, bring about sleepiness; and the tranquilizers, as a group, slow down reaction and movement time. Older people are already slowing down without any help from tranquilizer drugs.

As a result we have run a series of experiments in the lab to test the tranquilizing effect of exercise. In these experiments we found a very significant tranquilizer effect with young subjects, with middle-aged subjects, and with older subjects—older being of an average age of about 70. Not only did we get immediate or acute effects, but we also found chronic effects. In other words, training over a period of time resulted in a better ability to relax, as well as improving all these other functions.

We also found in the different experiments that many different kinds of exercise are effective. We got results from walking, from jogging, from cycling, and from bench stepping; thus apparently the type of exercise is not so important as is continuing it for 15 or 20 minutes, and not letting it become too intense. We find that a brisk 15-minute walk best accomplishes the goal.

A study we did at Leisure World (in southern California) looked at five treatment conditions. We had complete controls where the individual simply came in and spent his time in the lab for 30 minutes. We used meprobamate, the active ingredient in Miltown and Equanil, which at that time were the most popular tranquilizing drugs prescribed. A placebo and meprobamate were administered double blind, and then we administered a walking-type exercise at heart rate 100 and an exercise at heart rate 120. Each subject was his own control, so it was a fairly powerful test. There is a significant difference among those five treatments at the $\leq .01$ level, meaning that it is not likely that these data came about by chance.

First of all, there was no significant difference when comparing either the placebo or the meprobamate against controls. That is not to say that meprobamate is not effective as a tranquilizer. It is, but you have to take it for 2 or 3 days at two or three dosages per day before you begin achieving an effect that shows on electromyography.

There is no acute effect from one dose of meprobamate, whereas the exercise at heart rate 100 brought about a 20% reduction in tension. This was significant at the ≤ .01 level, also not likely due to chance.

Thus I believe it is important to realize that exercise provides an excellent tranquilizing effect. Incidentally, the data for walking at heart rate 120 were much less consistent and consequently did not achieve significance. What we believe happened is that a heart rate of 120 became for some people somewhat stressful; the resulting catecholamine response defeats our purpose, of course. Our best guess at this point, therefore, is that we need to keep the exercise moderate; we define moderate as 15 or 20 minutes of merely brisk walking. Overly vigorous exercise is definitely counterproductive.

In conclusion, we should observe some sensible precautions that are necessary if we are going to use vigorous exercise. I usually define the term vigorous exercise as anything that takes us above 40% of the heart rate range. Careful progression is important; in other words, the individual must start at a level that is easy for him/her to achieve. It is very important to use careful warmup procedures.

Now for jogging, or other exercise of this sort, the jogging itself is the best warmup you can use. And over a period of time we have come to use jogging first, and then the calisthenics, rather than vice versa as we did at Laguna Hills for administrative purposes. From the physiological standpoint there is no better warmup than brisk walking or jogging; going into the calisthenics after having warmed up carefully is a much safer procedure.

Equally important with the warmup is the cooldown at the end of the exercise. At the end of a vigorous exercise workout such as jogging, it is very important to cool down gradually. (There is no concern about cooling down from walking.) In other words, do not just stop jogging and stand there. Your muscle pump has now quit working for you, so you are not getting enough blood back to your head; thus you might very possibly faint and fall. The appropriate follow up to any kind of vigorous workout is walking sufficient to bring your heart rate back down close to normal. We like to use the static stretching exercises following all vigorous calisthenics, or any kind of vigorous exercise, to prevent muscle problems. We have found them to be very effective.

In all of my professional life, the most satisfying and rewarding experience I have had was seeing the great improvements that we were able to bring about in these older men and women at Laguna Hills, California.

INDEX